# The Assessment of Aphasia
# and Related Disorders

# The Assessment of Aphasia and Related Disorders

## HAROLD GOODGLASS, Ph.D.

*with the collaboration of*

## EDITH KAPLAN, Ph.D.

*Boston Veterans Administration Hospital
and
Boston University Aphasia Research Center
Department of Neurology
Boston University School of Medicine*

*Second Edition*

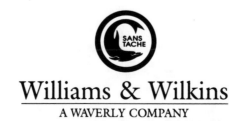

## Williams & Wilkins
### A WAVERLY COMPANY

BALTIMORE • PHILADELPHIA • LONDON • PARIS • BANGKOK
BUENOS AIRES • HONG KONG • MUNICH • SYDNEY • TOKYO • WROCLAW

Williams & Wilkins
Rose Tree Corporate Center, Building II
1400 North Providence Road, Suite 5025
Media, PA 19063-2043 USA

| | |
|---|---|
| First edition | 1972 |
| Reprinted | 1976 |
| Reprinted | 1978 |
| Reprinted | 1979 |
| Reprinted | 1981 |
| Reprinted | 1982 |
| Second edition | 1983 |
| Reprinted | 1994 |
| Reprinted | 1996 |

**Complete package includes:**

Harold Goodglass and Edith Kaplan:
    *The Assessment of Aphasia and Related Disorders*, 2nd ed.
*Boston Diagnostic Aphasia Examination Booklet* (32 pages)†
*Test Stimulus Cards* (16 cards)
*Boston Naming Test* (64 pages)
*Boston Naming Test Scoring Booklet* (8 pages)

†One copy bound in book after page 102 of the text.

**Additional materials (NOT RETURNABLE) available from Williams & Wilkins only:**
*Boston Diagnostic Aphasia Examination Booklet* (32 pages) (in multiples of 25):
        25—$23.00, *50*—$46.00,
        *75*—$69.00, *100*—$92.00.
*Test Stimulus Cards* (16 cards) at $9.50 per set.*
*Boston Naming Test* (64 pages) at $13.50 each.
*Boston Naming Test Scoring Booklet* (8 pages) (in multiples of 25):
        25—$12.00, *50*—$24.00,
        *75*—$36.00, *100*—$48.00

* Payment by check, Master Card, VISA, or American Express must accompany orders for Test
  Stimulus Cards when ordered separately from other available materials.

Williams & Wilkins, Rose Tree Corporate Center, Building II, 1400 North Providence Road, Suite 5025, Media, PA 19063-2043 USA

**Library of Congress Cataloging in Publication Data**

Goodglass, Harold.
    The assessment of aphasia and related disorders.

    Bibliography: p.
    Includes index.
    1. Aphasia—Diagnosis. I. Kaplan, Edith, 1924–
II. Title. [DNLM: 1. Aphasia. 2. Speech disorders.
WL 340.5 G651a]
RC425.G66   1984      616.85'52      83-9326
ISBN 0-8121-0901-5

Printed in the United States of America

Print number:   15  14  13  12  11

# Preface

World War II marked the beginning of a reawakening of interest in aphasia that has continued unabated until now. The immediate stimuli for this interest were the presence of large numbers of brain-injured, speech-disabled soldiers and the social obligation to rehabilitate them. Immediately on the heels of the postwar era came the burgeoning of activities related to the rehabilitation of the handicapped, particularly victims of stroke and head injury, of whom the aphasics make up an important segment. In response to this growth, the training of speech clinicians increased tremendously and, concurrently, the neuropsychologic study of normal and pathologic brain function attracted many able researchers.

A further and predictable response to these circumstances was the appearance on the market of a number of manuals on aphasia and aphasia testing. The earliest and most widely used was Eisenson's *Examining for Aphasia* (1954), followed by the Wepman and Jones *Language Modalities Test for Aphasia* (1961) and Schuell's *Differential Diagnosis of Aphasia with the Minnesota Test* (1965). In the area of childhood language disturbances, the McCarthy and Kirk *Illinois Test of Psycholinguistic Abilities* (1966) met wide acceptance.

Why, then, the need for another manual and test for aphasia? The principal answer is that the authors of the present work believe it offers features that give the examiner more insight into the patient's functioning and that serve as a bridge to relating test scores to the common aphasic syndromes recognized by neurologists. The Boston Diagnostic Aphasia Examination was developed in a center in which the rehabilitation of aphasics is part of a multidisciplinary approach, along with the study of the neuropathologic correlates of the varieties of aphasia and the psycholinguistic analysis of aphasic language. The test inevitably reflects the converging interests of these disciplines.

The opening two chapters of the manual present the authors' orientation to the nature of aphasic disorders and the goals and rationale of the assessment procedure. While an effort is made to place this discussion in the context of the history and relevant current research on aphasia, it is by no means intended as a comprehensive review of either history or research. The third chapter cites the statistical data available up to the present time. Chapter 4 describes the test procedure, subtest by subtest, and is intended to serve as an instruction manual for the examiner. Chapter 5 describes additional, unstandardized, special language testing procedures, some of which are being investigated experimentally and others that are used informally at the center. Chapter 6 describes a supplementary nonverbal battery covering apraxia and the quantitative, visuospatial, and somatognostic problems that, in addition to language, are so often implicated.

Finally, Chapter 7 describes the major aphasic syndromes as well as some of the rare "pure" forms of selective aphasia and shows how each pattern is reflected in the Aphasia Test score profile, with the help of selected case summaries.

In the 11 years since the publication of the

first edition, we have learned more about aphasia, both from clinical experience and through formal research. We have also had the benefit of critical comments about our aphasia examination and how it might be improved. Much of this experience and criticism is reflected in the revised text and test booklet.

From the point of view of diagnosis and brain localization, we have come through the era of the computerized tomographic (CT) scan, which has added immeasurably to our knowledge of relationships between language symptomatology and brain lesions. Studies with the CT scan have made us aware of the frequency of purely subcortical infarctions and hemorrhages and of configurations of language deficits associated with such lesions. Although syndromes of subcortical aphasias are not yet as clearly defined as the classic syndromes of cortical aphasia, they have some features that are discussed in the final chapter. If the first edition appeared to suggest that there is a limited set of "real" syndromes of aphasia corresponding to specific cortical foci, we have attempted, in this revision, to reverse that implication. The usefulness of the concept of well-defined syndromes, nevertheless, is as great as ever, as is the identification of the dimensions of language performance that characterize these syndromes.

Among the criticisms we have had of the Aphasia Examination itself, none involved major test revisions. Only a few (and very minor) changes, therefore, have been made in the test procedure. These consist in the reordering of some items within subtests and the addition of three body part names to the Confrontation Naming subtest, along with the elimination of the Body-Part Naming subtest. Significant changes have been made in the organization of the test record booklet; among them, a new subtest summary page, computed on the basis of percentiles instead of z-scores. Thus, the user of the examination may continue to use the existing stimulus materials, since all revisions are contained in the test record book.

Norms have been recomputed on a new sample of 242 aphasic subjects, and norms for neurologically normal adults are now included in the text.

This edition is accompanied by the Boston Naming Test, a wide-range picture naming-vocabulary test, which is often a valuable supplement to the Boston Diagnostic Aphasia Examination and which has useful application in the examination of children with learning disabilities and in the neuropsychologic evaluation of brain-injured adults.

A number of our collaborators deserve special thanks. The authors' theoretic orientation has been influenced by the late Dr. Fred A. Quadfasel, former Chief of Neurology at Boston Veterans Administration Hospital, and by Dr. Norman Geschwind, Professor of Neurology at Harvard Medical School. Dr. Robin Morris of Georgia State University is responsible for the factor analyses of the Boston Diagnostic Aphasia Examination and for the discriminant function analysis applied to the scores of selected prototypical representatives of the four major syndromes. Dr. Nancy Helm-Estabrooks, Chief of the Audiology and Speech Pathology Section, and her staff provided many valuable suggestions based on their long experience with the Boston Diagnostic Aphasia Examination. In particular, Patricia Fitzpatrick and Barbara Barresi collaborated in the amendment of the scales for assessing the Mechanics of Writing and Narrative Writing. Dr. Mary R. Hyde was invaluable to us in carrying out the data processing and providing collaboration with Dr. Robin Morris. Drs. Joan Borod and Carol Biber have seen to the accuracy and up-to-dateness of the computer files of all of our patients' scores. Jean C. Theurkauf did the artwork involved in displaying patients' performance graphically. We are also grateful to Roger Ray and Mrs. Betty Norky for sharing the typing of multiple drafts of this work.

The work on the revision of this examination was supported by Grants NS 06209 and NS 07615 from the National Institute of Neurological and Communicative Disorders and Stroke. The data for the revision could not have been obtained without the clinical facilities and patients of the Aphasia-Neurobehavior Unit of Boston Veterans Administration Medical Center.

*Boston, Massachusetts*    HAROLD GOODGLASS, Ph.D.

EDITH KAPLAN, Ph.D.

# Contents

# CHAPTER 1

# *Background*

The modern history of aphasia is usually dated back to the ferment over Broca's presentation of evidence for the localization of motor aphasia in the *Bulletin de la Société d'anthropologie* in 1861. The phenomenon of loss of speech due to brain injury is as old as recorded medicine, however, and Benton's review (1964) establishes that virtually all of the currently recognized aphasic symptoms were described long before the nineteenth century. The three decades preceding Broca's historic contribution witnessed increasing interest and controversy over the mechanisms of organic language disorders (Hécaen and Dubois, 1969), so that the events of 1861 fell on fertile ground.

It was only with the work of Broca, Wernicke, and their contemporaries, however, that certain organic impairments of language functions were finally grouped together under the term "aphasia" and recognized as distinct from the other intellectual impairments that might accompany them as byproducts of cerebral damage. The almost exclusive association of language loss with injury to a portion of the left cerebral hemisphere was recognized during the 1860s and the concept of unilateral cerebral dominance thus arose. Moreover, within a few decades of Broca's first localizing discoveries, it became clear that certain specific patterns of language loss could be reliably assigned to lesions in specific regions *within* the language area. The fascinating history of these discoveries and the nineteenth-century theories about the neurologic organization of language are reported in the classic works by Head (1926) and Weisenburg and McBride (1935) and in recent historical papers by Benton (1964) and Geschwind (1966).

The examination protocols of these neurologists, as detailed in their clinical reports, often reveal thorough inventories of language performance in all modalities. Moreover, since these workers were often sophisticated in problems of language, they paid attention to many of the more subtle aspects of aphasic language disorders and included analyses of grammar and syntax in their case studies.

In this presentation, we propose to continue in the tradition of approaching the aphasia examination as a psychologic analysis and measurement of language-related skills on one hand and, on the other hand, as a problem in relating particular configurations of symptoms with their neuropathologic correlates.

## THE PURPOSES OF APHASIA TESTING

The examination for aphasia may be geared to any one of three general aims: (1) diagnosis of presence and type of aphasic syndrome, leading to inferences concerning cerebral localization; (2) measurement of the level of performance over a wide range, for both initial determination and detection of change over time; (3) comprehensive assessment of the assets and liabilities of the patient in all language areas as a guide to therapy.

It is possible to design tests that perform any one of these functions well but fall short in one or both of the others. The present test is designed to meet all three of these applications, making it maximally useful to the

1

neurologist, the psychologist, the speech pathologist, and the speech therapist.

The diagnostic aim is met by a comprehensive sampling of all the variables in language performance that have proven useful in identifying the aphasic syndromes. We have attempted to make each subtest procedure as independent as possible of contaminating factors, recognizing that there is virtually no factorially pure test. Thus, the examination explicitly investigates seriatim speech, repetition, word production, and word comprehension in such special semantic categories as objects, actions, body parts, colors, letters, and numbers. Further, by means of rating scales and error classification the examiner is directed to those features of language that are not readily reduced to pass-fail scores, but that are of critical importance in arriving at a diagnostic decision. These include speech melody, fluency, anomia, syntactic organization, and the various forms of paraphasia.

The measurement function embodies certain requirements that are met in this test. These requirements are: (1) wide range of difficulty, (2) adequate subtest length for reliability and for discrimination of change, and (3) standardization to provide an external reference point of degrees of severity in each area tested.

The survey of the aphasic patient's assets and liabilities is made by comparing the effectiveness of various alternative ways of eliciting speech, comprehension, reading, and writing. Not only is the survey exceptionally complete, but the availability of percentile scores for each subtest frees the examiner from purely impressionistic judgments about the patient's relative impairment in one area as compared to another.

### Limitations

The limitations of this test battery are those that are inherent in any aphasia test. The materials and procedures provided by the test merely serve as convenient aids for sampling relevant performances of the patient. This sampling is not exhaustive, and the examiner should feel free to introduce variations on the standard procedures to further explore avenues suggested by the errors of a particular patient. The scores do not objectively and automatically classify the patient, nor do they point to an optimum approach to therapy. The greater the experience of the examiner, the more useful the interpretations that can be made from the test record. The case illustrations will serve as a guide but not as a source of cookbook formulas for diagnosis.

## PRINCIPLES UNDERLYING THIS EXAMINATION

The design of this Aphasia Test is based on the observation that various components of language may be selectively damaged by aphasia and that this selectivity is a clue to (1) the anatomic organization of language in the brain, (2) the localization of the causative lesion, and (3) the functional interactions of various parts of the language system.

It must be pointed out that the foregoing position is not universally accepted. Schuell, Jenkins and Jiménez-Pabón (1964), for example, attribute most of the significant variations among aphasia subtests to impairment of general language capacity. There are many factors in the aphasia testing situation that tend to erase the evidence for any underlying independence of components in language:

1. It is difficult to devise a single task that can be passed or failed through only one process.
2. Though the various neural subsystems of language may be selectively vulnerable at certain anatomic points, they are almost certainly intermingled in other areas of the left hemisphere. The larger the lesion in these areas, the greater the effect on many functions.
3. The bulk of the clinical material for quantitative studies comes from cases in which large lesions are the rule, implicating, simultaneously, functionally diverse areas. Small lesions producing isolated disorders occur less frequently and therefore have a smaller effect in any study that groups all cases together.
4. The usual distribution of severity of aphasics in hospitals, as Schuell points out, is bimodal, with many severe and residual aphasics but few at intermedi-

ate levels. This spread overemphasizes the severity factor, producing large intercorrelations and obscuring differences in process between tasks.

If all language performance in aphasia were merely a function of the status of "general language ability," the ideal aphasia test would consist of a handful of tasks most highly loaded on this factor, which would be presumed to predict fairly well the standing on all other tests. Alternatively, we might settle for a general communication score. We accept the usefulness of these global measures, but hold that there is also much more to be learned from an aphasia examination.

Returning to the construction of the present test, we tried first to assess the components of language as nearly as possible in isolated form. It is impossible to reach this ideal completely, since one can test an expressive function only by choosing some instrumental input channel through which to elicit the expressive behavior. In the same way, one can test receptive functions only by designating an instrumental response modality through which the subject demonstrates his comprehension. Generally, we regard the instrumental modality as only one of several possible "windows" on the capacity in question. If the validity of the view through one "window" is in doubt, we improvise another, if it is not already provided by the test. We specifically reject the view of language as being based primarily on a collection of stimulus-response systems. In this respect, our approach is different from that of Wepman's *Language Modalities Test for Aphasia* (1961).

For example, desiring to know how a patient appreciates oral spelling, we choose the response mode or "window" of having him tell us orally what we have spelled for him. If his speech production is much impaired, it provides a clouded "window," and we must find another approach to assess his comprehension of orally spelled words—perhaps multiple-choice selection of pictures to correspond with the spelled word (not provided in the test). To take another example, if we wish to test the word-finding ability of a patient, we may approach it through the instrumental mode of showing him objects visually,

or we may have him feel them tactually or listen to the sounds they make or answer questions requiring their names. Each of these "windows" on word-finding has its own characteristics as a receptive modality that make it more or less effective as a means of eliciting the desired response. Studies by Spreen, Benton, and Van Allen (1966) and by Goodglass, Barton, and Kaplan (1968) show that, with few exceptions, aphasics name objects equally well through whatever sensory modality they are presented. The concept of independent stimulus-response channels going directly from each modality-specific receptive system to the oral output system is not supported. The few instances of modality-specific naming defects are of great interest, but where anatomic information is available it indicates isolation of the sensory input from the entire left cerebral language system.

In playing down the role of stimulus-response units in language, we argue that the vast bulk of functional language behavior involves either self-initiated linguistic output or responses in which it is apparent that complex intermediary steps have occurred between the perception of a linguistic or other sensory input and the output. The immediate response to a linguistic stimulus is an implicit one that we can assess only indirectly through the test performance that we choose. There are a number of elementary language skills that do not require comprehension or formulation of a meaningful message, however, that may be defended as stimulus-response units. These are, for the most part, direct imitations of the input, as in the case of repetition of spoken language or copying of written language. Even in these cases, we must assure ourselves that the receptive process and the output capability are intact before considering a performance failure to be a loss of the stimulus-response unit. For example, it may be shown that oral repetition can break down in the presence of intact auditory comprehension and considerable fluency of spontaneous or conversational speech.

Can the same be said for copying written language in cases in which copying is the only means of eliciting a patient's writing? In most cases—especially when the patient can transcribe—we are probably dealing with a direct evocation of writing movements in response to seeing letters. When all means of recalling writing have been lost, the patient may still copy slavishly, but he is now calling on his general ability to reproduce simple geometric forms.

In summary, then, the subtests of the battery in most cases represent alternative "windows" that enable us to infer the status of an underlying capacity. In a few cases, they are direct samples of a stimulus-response unit that usually represents one of the elementary language performance skills.

CHAPTER 2

# *The Nature of the Deficits*

Normal language may be regarded as depending on a complex interaction between sensory-motor skills, symbolic associations, and habituated syntactic patterns, all at the service of the speaker's intent to communicate, and subject to the intellectual capacity that he brings to the task of manipulating them so as to carry out his intent. Aphasia refers to the disturbance of any or all of the skills, associations, and habits of spoken or written language produced by injury to certain brain areas that are specialized for these functions. Disturbances of language usage that are due to paralysis or incoordination of the musculature of speech or writing or to poor vision or hearing or to severe intellectual impairment are not, of themselves, aphasic. Such disorders may accompany an aphasia, however, and thus complicate the clinical manifestations of the language defect proper.

A century of intensive analysis of aphasic symptoms has produced considerable agreement as to identifiable component deficits, some of which may appear in some cases in nearly pure form, and, in others, may stand out by their severity on a background of milder impairment in the remaining language skills. Thus, one may find extreme, selective disorders of auditory comprehension, object-naming, articulation, reading, or repetition, to give a few instances. Not only is there wide consensus as to the individual component deficits to be observed, but the common clusters of defects (i.e., the major aphasic syndromes) emerge repeatedly in the interpretive observations of dozens of careful writers, though often under different names based on different theoretic biases.

The deficits of aphasia and their common clustering in general cannot be deduced by a logical analysis of the normal speech process; they are empirically derived. The subtests of this aphasia battery have, in turn, been chosen so as to elicit quantitive evidence of the many possible specific areas of deficit. Where objective quantification is not feasible, the examiner is provided with rating scales.

## ENUMERATION OF AREAS OF DEFICIT

### Articulation

Patients with the most severe articulatory disorders are unable voluntarily to produce simple sounds, even by imitation. Each effort may end up with the emission of the same, recurrent word or nonsense syllable, often to the chagrin of the patient. In somewhat milder form, the patient may be considerably aided by imitation, but may articulate laboriously, with distortions of the more difficult sounds, particularly consonant blends. Vowels tend to return to normal earlier than do consonants. Success in finding the articulatory movement sequences for a given word is often an all-or-none affair. As the patient improves, he may pronounce common words and phrases normally, but may experience severe articulatory difficulty with less common words.

Articulatory difficulty, as an aphasic component, is distinguished from nonaphasic dysarthria by its variability. The aphasic often reveals perfectly normal articulation during automatized sequences (e.g., counting) or in repeating, or in exclaiming. Increased effort may only aggravate his difficulty. A nonaphasic dysarthria is more constant under all conditions and may be somewhat controlled by attention and effort on the patient's part.

Because the task of repetition often masks the articulatory difficulty of aphasics, this standard approach to testing articulation is not used here. Instead, the present examination relies on articulation ratings for each response in a variety of speech tasks, as well as on an articulation rating scale.

## Loss of Verbal Fluency

The ability to produce words in connected sequences is closely associated with ease of articulation, but is not *always* predicted by articulation. That is, patients who pronounce individual words clearly may go through a separate effort to emit each word or, at best, produce short word groupings with each separate effort. More rarely, poor articulation may be compatible with considerable fluency. Fluency is best rated in terms of the longest occasional uninterrupted strings of words that are produced. It has been found to be reliably ratable in this way and to be an important diagnostic criterion (Goodglass, Quadfasel, and Timberlake, 1964).

Fluency is best judged from speech production during extended conversation and free narrative. The present examination procedure prescribes an interview, followed by presentation of a complex picture situation as a stimulus for a short narrative description. A rating scale for fluency is included in a set of six rating scales for those speech characteristics that are difficult to quantify objectively.

## Word-Finding Difficulty

Virtually all aphasics suffer some restriction in the repertory of words that they have available for speech and require increased time to produce these words. For most patients, the frequent words of the language are the first to be recovered and are produced with the briefest delay. In some patients, however, loss of the power to evoke words corresponding to specific concepts is disproportionately severe as compared to the level of fluency and articulation. These patients show a striking inability to name even common objects, action words, colors, adjectives, and other categories of words. There is a subtle qualitative difference between the general restriction of vocabulary, common to most aphasics, and the selective loss of the ability to evoke specific words, which is called "word-finding difficulty" or "anomia."

Since patients with anomia are usually relatively fluent in producing a flow of small talk or rambling uninformative speech, it has been noted that their speech sounds "empty," that is, lacking in the critical words necessary to convey meaning.

The obvious way of testing word-finding difficulty would seem to be to present pictures or questions requiring the selection of a particular word in response. This test approach by itself fails, however, to distinguish the anomic patient from the patient who cannot articulate or from the patient with a generalized severe restriction of speech. One of the common features of anomia is the selectivity shown among categories of words. Nouns are the most severely impaired category, whereas many patients retain their ability to name letters and numbers (Goodglass, Klein, Carey, and Jones, 1966). We have made a special point, therefore, of sampling each of several word categories.

The decision as to whether word-finding difficulty is a diagnostically discriminating significant feature of an aphasic's speech pattern, therefore, cannot be made from a correctness count on any single test, but rather depends on the pattern observed in conversation. Here again, we provide a rating scale to be applied to the sample of conversation and narrative speech.

## Repetition

The ability to reproduce, from auditory presentation, patterns of familiar speech sounds is normally acquired early in life and is one of the most elementary mechanisms at the core of spoken language. Mentally defective persons who have little capacity to convey or understand information through language may have this particular sensory-motor system intact, so that they can echo speech and can acquire passages by rote.

Repetition in aphasia may be disturbed at three points in the process. First, the patient may fail at the level of recognition. He may fail to grasp the sounds as words and, consequently, refuse to attempt to repeat them, or he may capture only certain fragments of the spoken model. Second, he may fail at the level of articulation in spite of his ability to demonstrate that he knows the meaning of the test words or sentence. Finally, he may fail because of a selective dissociation between auditory input and the speech-output system. The latter group of patients may demonstrate fairly fluent speech and near-perfect comprehension, yet have extraordinary difficulty in repeating what they have heard. This difficulty is increased by the length and unfamiliarity of the material to be repeated, and it depends as well on the grammatical composition of the sentence. In this aphasia examination, tests for repetition of words as well as for sentences of increasing length are included.

Not only is the selective impairment of repetition diagnostically significant, but also its selective retention in an otherwise severe aphasia.

## Seriatim Speech

It has long been observed that the recitation of memorized sequences (e.g., counting, days of the week) may be partially spared in severely aphasic patients of all types. Thus, although these items are almost always included in aphasia tests, they rarely are diagnostically important for distinguishing between varieties of aphasics. An occasional patient who may otherwise be bereft of useful speech will show extraordinary retention of the ability to recite, not only the familiar word series, but even poetry or long prayers. This configuration is particularly notable when associated with good repetition. Like repetition, the ability to reel off a memorized sequence represents the operation of an elementary sensory-motor skill of spoken language that says nothing about the ability to associate meaning to the spoken word, either receptively or expressively.

In this aphasia examination, the performance of automatized speech is sampled through the usual tasks of reciting numbers, days, months, and the alphabet, as well as nursery rhymes.

## Loss of Grammar and Syntax

Clinically, one observes that some aphasics are totally lacking in the ability to place words together in grammatically organized sequences, while other patients, equally disabled in effective speech, may have great facility in framing sentences of many varieties.

The term "agrammatism" is used to describe the speech of patients who can juxtapose some nouns and verbs to convey a message, but who omit virtually all the small grammatical words and inflectional markers of verb tense, person, and number. The milder form of this disorder, "telegraphic speech," denotes partial availability of sentence forms, but with deletion of many articles, prepositions, conjunctions, auxiliary verbs, and inflectional endings. In most instances, patients with either telegraphic or agrammatic speech are nonfluent, often with impaired articulation, stemming from lesions in the anterior speech zone of the left hemisphere.

Note that the disorder entails omission of grammatical connectives and indicators of relations between words, and simplification to short phrases and sentences. Agrammatism is not to be confused with "paragrammatism," in which *most* inflections and small grammatical words fall smoothly into place, but with unsystematic substitutions or omissions of both grammatical morphemes and lexical words (i.e., nouns, verbs, adjectives), and tangled grammatical organization. In contrast to the nonfluent delivery of agrammatic and telegraphic speech, paragrammatic patients are fluent or even "hyperfluent," in that their output is often rapid and resistant to interruptions. Paragrammatism is associated classically with lesions of the posterior speech zones, notably Wernicke's aphasia.

Patients who are agrammatic in speech production commonly show similar problems in their attempts to repeat sentences, in their oral reading, and in their writing. Agrammatic features may, however, be confined to a single output channel (Miceli et al., 1983; Goodglass and Menn, in press).

The comprehension of syntactic relations in auditorily presented sentences and in silent reading may be impaired in aphasic patients, regardless of whether they speak agrammatically. There is some evidence in the literature, however, that patients with agrammatic speech are more prone to ignore grammatical morphemes in their reading than are fluent aphasics (von Stockert and Bader, 1976).

Although the identification of agrammatism and of paragrammatism is vital for diagnostic purposes, there are no satisfactory objective tests to measure the grammatical dimension in speech output. It is clear that simply counting grammatical errors will not discriminate between these diametrically opposite symptoms, which are indicators of widely different lesion sites. In this version of our aphasia examination, we therefore continue the former practice of relying on a rating scale for "variety of grammatical forms available" to identify the presence and severity of agrammatism, and another scale for the rating of "paraphasia in running speech," which is sensitive to the presence of paragrammatism.

The value of specifically examining the *comprehension* of particular syntactic arrangements as an aid in diagnosis or in the assessment of auditory or written language comprehension has not been established. Subtests for the comprehension of spoken and written sentences and paragraphs, which are included in this examination, do not separate the syntactic from the lexical aspects of sentence comprehension. We therefore continue to provide tests aimed specifically at syntactic comprehension in the chapter on supplementary tests.

### Paraphasia

Paraphasia refers to the production of unintended syllables, words, or phrases during the effort to speak. In general, paraphasia is characteristic of patients whose speech sounds are uttered fluently. The distorted pronunciation of patients with poor articulation does *not* come under this heading.

Under the rubric of paraphasia, the following specific varieties are diagnostically distinctive:

LITERAL (OR PHONEMIC) PARAPHASIA. In spite of easy articulation of individual sounds, the patient produces syllables in the wrong order or distorts his words with unintended sounds. For example, "pipe" may become "Hike . . . no, pike . . . pipe!" Some phonemic features (usually the vowels and the number of syllables) of the intended words are preserved, thus distinguishing literal paraphasic utterances from complete neologisms. When words are grossly distorted with literal paraphasia, we use the term *neologistic distortion,* an extreme literal paraphasic error.

VERBAL PARAPHASIA. When an unintended word is inadvertently used in place of another, the substituted words are usually related in connotative sphere (e.g., "my mother" in place of "my wife") to the intended word. These may be referred to as "semantic paraphasias" as opposed to "remote paraphasia," in which the substitution seems totally capricious, or as opposed to "perseverative paraphasia," in which the word used crops up again from something said just previously. Verbal paraphasias, which are *unintended,* should be distinguished from "one-word circumlocutions," in which the patient deliberately chooses an approximation to his intended idea because of his word-finding difficulty (e.g., he substitutes the word, "Chesterfield," for "cigarette").

PARAGRAMMATISM OR EXTENDED PARAPHASIA. This refers to running speech that is logically incoherent either because the phrases do not make sense together or because of intrusions of misused words, neologisms, or all of these features. One may not be able to identify specific word substitutions that would qualify as verbal paraphasias.

SCORING OF PARAPHASIA. In this examination, each instance of paraphasia is tallied as it occurs during the testing. Separate columns are provided for literal, neologistic, verbal, and extended paraphasia. The relative frequency of the various types of paraphasia is reflected in the Subtest Summary Profile sheet. In addition, the occurrence of paraphasia in running speech is rated on the Profile of Speech Characteristics.

### Auditory Comprehension

Disturbances of auditory comprehension may take various forms, with varying degrees of severity in each aspect. The present battery measures some, but not all, of these dimensions. For example, a most dramatic, but uncommon, form of comprehension defect is "word-deafness," in which the patient reacts *as though* he has not heard the words spoken to him or has captured only fragments of their sounds. On repeated presentation, he may succeed in grasping the sounds and then, at once, understand the word. More commonly (as seen in Wernicke's aphasia), the defect does not involve the recognition of sounds, but rather the association of meaning to them, for the patient may repeat aloud, uncomprehendingly, words spoken to him. Although both these forms of disorder may produce the same objective test score, their clinical manifestations are clearly different.

In particular, Wernicke's aphasics are often strikingly worse in grasping words in isolation than in a sentence context. They benefit from the additional clues to meaning that they garner from the rest of the sentence. Thus, length of utterance does not increase difficulty of comprehension in a simple linear fashion. It is only when length is combined with the demand to grasp multiple significant informational elements that comprehension suffers.

When auditory comprehension is only partially impaired, the patient's success may depend on the familiarity of the words used, on the length and informational density of the message and on the intellectual simplicity of the message to be understood. In this battery, we examine for *comprehension vocabulary* by means of a "word-discrimination" subtest of single words; we examine capacity for information by means of commands of increasing length; we examine intellectual grasp by means of a set of "yes"-"no" questions demanding increasing powers of inference about questions of fact, but not beyond the capacity of average adults.

Further, recognizing that words of a given semantic class may be selectively affected, we divide the word-discrimination test into "objects," "actions," "colors," "numbers," "letters," "geometric shapes," and "body parts." The chapter on supplementary language tests provides a section on whole body commands (e.g., "Stand up, turn around, walk backwards, and return to your seat."). Paradoxically, these are often well preserved.

Currently under study is the difficulty of grasping certain grammatical words and grammatical constructions, such as prepositional relationships and instances in which meaning depends on word order (e.g., "my brother's wife" vs. "my wife's brother"). These may be severely impaired in patients who have excellent word discrimination, yet unaccountably fail to grasp certain commands. Thus, the present battery does not deprive the examiner of the opportunity to improvise and explore the patient's capacity. The examiner must take into account the easy fatigability of comprehension, failures brought about by difficulty in shifting between topics, and the facilitating effect of making the conversation personally relevant to the patient.

## Reading

The normal acquisition of reading appears to be based on the prior mastery of auditory language, and evidence from aphasia supports the concept that the neurologic basis of reading includes the auditory comprehension system, in addition to structures that provide an association between the auditory and the visual processes. Thus, aphasias involving severe impairment of auditory language almost invariably impair reading—particularly reading of connected material. The most striking apparent exception to this rule is in the case of pure word-deafness (described previously), in which reading is preserved. The anatomic reason proposed for this exception is that the auditory association area is essentially intact, but disconnected from its input from the primary auditory areas.

The relation between reading and auditory comprehension levels is often confusing in the Wernicke's aphasic. These patients, as we have observed, may fail to grasp a word that is spoken to them out of context, even while repeating it correctly. On seeing the same word written, they often understand it at once. Thus, at the one-word level, reading is superior to auditory comprehension. When the written message increases to sentence length, its difficulty increases enormously, while comprehension of the spoken message is some-times facilitated by the sentence context.

May reading comprehension be autono-mous from the auditory comprehension sys-tem? We know that deaf-mutes learn to read and grasp meaning without ever having had an auditory experience of the word. It is plau-sible that this mode of reading plays at least a secondary role in normal reading, as well. It is a common observation that some aphasics grasp meaning while saying the wrong word aloud. Conversely, some patients will point to a written word related in meaning, but not in sound, to a spoken model.

A group of aphasic patients have been iden-tified who have virtually complete loss of the ability to apply phonic rules to derive sound from spelling, i.e., they have lost graphopho-nemic conversion rules. They often show an extreme degree of verbal paralexia, i.e., oral production of a semantically related but vis-ually unrelated rendition of a written word. Their ability to produce either correct or se-mantically related responses depends on the semantic meaningfulness and concreteness of the written word. They do best with pictur-able nouns and less well with verbs and ad-jectives; they fail totally to read aloud gram-matical morphemes or inflectional endings, as well as to read nonsense syllables. This dis-order, referred to as "deep dyslexia" (Mar-shall and Newcombe, 1973), has been studied extensively (Coltheart, Patterson and Mar-shall, 1980).

The analytic examination of reading re-quires determination of whether letters and words are recognized as familiar configura-tions, quite apart from their meaning. Can spoken and written words be matched on the basis of phonic associations, still without con-cern for meaning? Both of these functions are examined by means of multiple-choice sub-tests. In the rare cases of alexia caused purely by disconnection of the visual input from the cortical language area, the patient continues to understand oral spelling. Comprehension of oral spelling may be lost either because of impaired recognition or limited auditory span for letter names or because of disturbance of the audiovisual associations on which reading is based.

The simplest level of reading for meaning

is that of pairing written words with corre-sponding concepts, usually in the form of pic-tures. In our examination, a multiple-choice selection of pictures is used. Comprehension of connected text is then tested by means of a graded series of multiple-choice sentence completion items, increasing from three-word sentences to paragraph length.

## Writing

Writing is the most complex of the lan-guage modalities and has a correspondingly large number of dimensions for examination. At the level of mere motor execution, writing may fail with respect to the recall of the form of letters or of the movements involved in producing them. As in speech, there are auto-matized, serial tasks, such as writing one's name and address, or the alphabet, that may be preserved when all other writing is lost. Slavish copying from a printed model may still be possible when the subject cannot tran-scribe into cursive script.

Although, in the speaker's mind, the small-est significant units of oral speech are mor-phemes, when we deal with writing, on the other hand, letters have much more auton-omy. The recall of letters to dictation, there-fore, is tested prior to examining the ability to write words to dictation.

When a word is written to dictation, we do not know whether the process involved is pri-marily one of phonetic translation from sound to spelling or whether comprehension of the meaning of the word has played an inter-mediary role. When the patient is required to write the names of pictured objects, however, we know that the initiating process is the con-cept of the object and we are testing "written word-finding." Observation of the writing process and of patient's errors indicate that three types of association are at work. One is the automatic translation of sounds into the motor sequences for letters, following the phonic rules of the language; another is the recall of syllables and short words as complete graphic motor sequences, bolstered by a visual model of the word configurations; a third is the availability of oral spelling as a guide to writing. Because oral spelling is unhampered by the slowness of recalling and writing individual letters, we often find oral spelling a bit superior to written spelling to dictation. Only by specifically testing each process do we obtain an inkling as to how they are interacting in the patient's performance of a complex writing task.

As we raised the question about reading, we may ask how independent written expression is from formulated oral language. Is there a direct association between concept and written expression that does not go through the intermediary of auditorily formulated inner speech? The performance of aphasics indicates that such autonomous writing may occur at the one-word level, when, for example, a patient writes or spells orally a word that he cannot recall in speech. Further evidence is seen in patients who, on dictation of a given word, write another that is related in meaning, but not in sound (paragraphia). The vast preponderance of aphasic performance indicates, however, that writing is built on the

capacity to formulate spoken language. Thus, the ability to write may approach, but rarely exceed, the capacity to speak. As in the case of reading, the exception to this rule is in patients whose disorder is purely articulatory and apparently spares the speech formulation system.

The medium of writing does not provide the melodic and rhythmic sentence contour that helps the aphasic to organize his grammatical sequences and, particularly, to fit in the small connectives and inflectional forms. Because writing is a slower, word-by-word process, sentence writing makes a heavy demand on knowledge of grammatical rules and on retention of the string of projected words, along with recall of what has already been written. Consequently, grammar may be more primitive in written language than in speech.

In our aphasia examination, the writing of connected material is elicited by dictation and by presentation of a story-picture, which the patient is asked to describe in writing.

CHAPTER 3

# Statistical Background

An evaluation of the reliability of the subtests was undertaken by selecting protocols of 34 patients who were distributed as follows on degree of severity of aphasia:

| N | Level | Description |
|---|-------|-------------|
| 0 | 0 | No communication possible. |
| 11 | 1 | Communication possible only by examiner's questioning and guessing. |
| 6 | 2 | Patient carries share of conversation, but range of information exchanged is limited. |
| 7 | 3 | Speech is defective in form and content but patient can convey almost all ideas. |
| 6 | 4 | Obvious handicap is present, although speech is largely correct and there is no limitation on expression. |
| 4 | 5 | Residual aphasia with only subjective difficulties. |

The Kuder-Richardson method of determining subtest reliability was applied. The resulting reliability coefficients are listed in Table 1. The subtests for which reliability data are omitted are those that are not based on a series of scoreable items and hence are not appropriate for this reliability measure.

The reliability coefficients obtained indicate good internal consistency within subtests with respect to what the items are measuring. Reliability, in the sense of repeatability of results on retesting any patient, varies among aphasics to a degree rarely found in other types of patients. Some subjects have wide fluctuations in efficiency from day to day as well as fluctuations depending on time of day. Once recovery has stabilized, however, the majority of aphasics will, on retest, repeat their earlier performance fairly closely. For-

mal test retest data have not been obtained with this instrument.

## 1972 STANDARDIZATION

The classification of any aphasic symptom configuration depends on the relative preservation of performance in various areas. Subtests covering these various areas vary in length and in absolute level of difficulty. Only the most experienced clinician can have any confidence in judging relative degrees of impairment between, for example, a score on a

**Table 1. Reliability Coefficients of Subtests**

| | $r_{xx}$ |
|---|---|
| Auditory Comprehension | |
| Word Discrimination | .96 |
| Body-Part Identification | .68 |
| Commands | .91 |
| Complex Ideational Material | .89 |
| Oral Expression | |
| Oral Agility—Nonverbal | .83 |
| Oral Agility—Verbal | .89 |
| Automatized Sequences | .82 |
| Repetition of Words | .92 |
| Repetition of Phrases | |
| a. High Probability | .90 |
| b. Low Probability | .91 |
| Word Reading | .95 |
| Responsive Naming | .92 |
| Visual Confrontation Naming | .98 |
| Oral Sentence Reading | .94 |
| Understanding Written Language | |
| Symbol and Word Discrimination | .90 |
| Phonetic Association | |
| a. Word Recognition | .80 |
| b. Comprehension of Oral Spelling | .91 |
| Word-Picture Matching | .92 |
| Reading Sentences and Paragraphs | .90 |
| Writing | |
| Spelling to Dictation | .89 |
| Written Confrontation Naming | .92 |

10-item written spelling test and a score on a 36-item picture-naming test. Thus it was important to develop some method of weighting so as to make subtest scores comparable among themselves.

The basic methodologic problem is that one cannot be sure of the significance of a mean score for aphasics on any test because the distribution of degrees of severity of aphasia is not known and may be highly skewed. Since we have access only to that part of the aphasic population that comes to the hospital and stays for rehabilitation, we have no way of knowing how they compare to the population of all aphasics.

In order to circumvent this problem, we decided to assign our aphasics to the six clinically defined severity levels listed on page 12 and compute subtest z-scores independently for patients at each severity level above the lowest. This procedure yielded five z-score subtest profile charts, the appropriate one to be chosen according to the patient's severity level. We felt that the cumbersomeness of this procedure would be justified if different profiles resulted from similar combinations of scores for patients at different severity levels.

Plotting of a number of patients' profiles on z-score charts based on severity groups other than their own did not significantly affect their profiles, other than to move them, intact, back or forth on the severity dimension. It was therefore decided that, for practical purposes, we could disregard the question of whether the distribution of our aphasic sample truly represented the population and proceed as though it did. The original score profile chart of the first (1972) edition was based on data from 207 patients at severity levels 1 through 5. Table 2 gives the range, mean, and standard deviation of the patients on each subtest in the 1972 sample and in the new sample.

## 1982 STANDARDIZATION

A revised score summary sheet (Figure 1) is introduced with the present revision, based on a new normative sample of 242 aphasics, tested at the Boston VA Medical Center between 1976 and 1982. In this revision, we have abandoned the standard score expressed as

z-scores in favor of percentiles. The use of percentiles as a means of converting raw scores on diverse subtests to a common scale has both a statistical and a practical advantage over z-scores. Statistically, unlike z-scores, percentiles are not affected by deviations from normality in the distribution of subtest scores. Many of the BDAE subtests yield highly skewed distributions. Practically, it is simpler to read a percentile scale: the gradations on the scale can be finer, and interpolation between the decile markings is easier. Moreover, the concept of percentiles is easier to grasp directly than that of z-scores. Z-scores must be understood in terms of standard deviations above and below a zero mean, while percentiles directly represent positions in the ranked population, in which the fiftieth percentile is the score falling at the median.

In the revised score summary sheet (Figure 1), we have changed the direction in which the four paraphasia scales are read. The number of paraphasias now is the inverse of the percentile rank, so that the most impaired (i.e., the highest paraphasia counts) fall in the lowest percentile, in keeping with all the other scores.

Because of factors affecting the selection of patients for admission to the Aphasia Unit at Boston VA Medical Center, the present sample has a greater proportion of selective aphasias, produced by a single vascular lesion than is found in many large rehabilitation programs. As compared to the 1972 sample, however, the representation of severe mixed aphasia (severity ratings of 0 or 1), produced by large lesions, is considerably greater because it includes test data on virtually every patient who passed through the unit. The difference in the makeup of the new normative sample undoubtedly affects both the intercorrelations between subtests and the structure of the factors derived from the intercorrelation matrix.

## CLUSTERING OF SUBTESTS*

Two approaches are taken to evaluate the interrelationships among the performances

---

*The collaboration of Robin Morris, Ph.D., in these analyses is gratefully acknowledged.

**Table 2.   Range, Mean, and Standard Deviation of Aphasics on Each Subtest; Comparison of 1972 and 1982 Samples**

| | 1972 | | | | 1982 | | | |
|---|---|---|---|---|---|---|---|---|
| | N | Range | M | SD | N | Range | M | SD |
| Severity Rating | 152 | 1–5 | 2.4 | 1.4 | 223 | 0–5 | 1.6* | 1.3 |
| Articulation Rating | 147 | 1–7 | 5.1 | 1.9 | 200 | 1–7 | 4.9 | .7 |
| Phrase-Length Rating | 147 | 1–7 | 5.2 | 2.0 | 207 | 1–7 | 4.4 | 2.5 |
| Paraphasia (Neologistic) | 180 | 0–10 | 1.8 | 6.7 | 201 | 0–40 | 5.0 | 7.9 |
| Paraphasia (Literal) | 180 | 0–29 | 3.1 | 5.0 | 200 | 0–47 | 7.2 | 8.1 |
| Paraphasia (Verbal) | 180 | 0–35 | 7.4 | 7.2 | 201 | 0–40 | 11.2 | 9.1 |
| Paraphasia (Extended) | 180 | 0–43 | 3.2 | 5.9 | 197 | 0–43 | 2.8 | 5.6 |
| Word Discrimination | 194 | 2–72 | 55.6 | 17.4 | 241 | 0–72 | 46.2 | 20.6 |
| Body-Part Identification | 195 | 0–20 | 14.2 | 5.8 | 241 | 0–20 | 12.1 | 6.6 |
| Commands | 193 | 0–15 | 10.2 | 5.2 | 240 | 0–15 | 9.0 | 4.6 |
| Complex Ideational Material | 192 | 0–12 | 6.6 | 4.0 | 241 | 0–12 | 5.2 | 3.7 |
| Verbal Agility | 191 | 0–14 | 8.1 | 4.6 | 198 | 0–14 | 7.5 | 4.9 |
| Nonverbal Agility | 183 | 0–12 | 5.2 | 3.1 | 97 | 0–12 | 6.8 | 3.4 |
| Automatized Sequences | 191 | 0–8 | 5.0 | 2.9 | 235 | 0–8 | 4.1 | 2.9 |
| Reciting | 186 | 0–2 | 0.8 | 0.8 | 224 | 0–2 | 0.9 | 0.8 |
| Singing | 183 | 0–2 | 1.3 | 0.8 | 225 | 0–2 | 1.6 | 0.7 |
| Rhythm | 186 | 0–2 | 1.0 | 0.8 | 222 | 0–2 | 1.3 | 0.7 |
| Repetition of Words | 192 | 0–10 | 7.3 | 3.3 | 238 | 0–10 | 6.1 | 3.6 |
| High-Probability Repetition | 187 | 0–8 | 3.9 | 3.2 | 240 | 0–8 | 3.0 | 3.0 |
| Low-Probability Repetition | 186 | 0–8 | 2.6 | 2.9 | 239 | 0–8 | 1.7 | 2.4 |
| Word Reading | 191 | 0–30 | 18.2 | 11.8 | 237 | 0–30 | 13.6 | 12.0 |
| Responsive Naming | 192 | 0–30 | 16.3 | 11.3 | 239 | 0–30 | 11.1 | 10.8 |
| Visual Confrontation Naming | 188 | 0–105 | 62.0 | 35.9 | 239 | 0–105 | 42.3* | 37.3 |
| Body-Part Naming | 50 | 0–30 | 17.0 | 11.1 | 233 | 0–30 | 11.3 | 10.2 |
| Animal Naming | 183 | 0–35 | 6.3 | 6.0 | 223 | 0–23 | 3.3 | 4.2 |
| Oral Sentence Reading | 187 | 0–10 | 4.6 | 3.6 | 234 | 0–10 | 2.8 | 3.5 |
| Symbol and Word Discrimination | 193 | 0–10 | 8.5 | 2.6 | 235 | 0–10 | 7.5 | 3.1 |
| Word Recognition | 193 | 0–8 | 6.3 | 2.2 | 235 | 0–8 | 5.3 | 2.5 |
| Comprehension of Oral Spelling | 193 | 0–8 | 3.4 | 3.1 | 228 | 0–8 | 2.4 | 2.7 |
| Word-Picture Matching | 192 | 0–10 | 7.5 | 3.2 | 234 | 0–10 | 6.1 | 3.8 |
| Reading Sentences and Paragraphs | 189 | 0–10 | 5.0 | 3.4 | 226 | 0–10 | 4.2 | 3.0 |
| Writing Mechanics | 191 | 0–3 | 2.3 | 1.0 | 232 | 0–3 | 2.2 | 0.9* |
| Serial Writing | 187 | 0–47 | 30.6 | 16.0 | 230 | 0–47 | 26.1 | 16.1 |
| Primer-Level Dictation | 187 | 0–15 | 9.8 | 5.5 | 231 | 0–15 | 7.8 | 5.6 |
| Spelling to Dictation | 184 | 0–10 | 3.7 | 2.9 | 218 | 0–10 | 2.3 | 2.8 |
| Written Confrontation Naming | 182 | 0–10 | 3.7 | 3.5 | 224 | 0–10 | 3.1 | 3.4 |
| Narrative Writing | 180 | 0–4 | 1.1 | 1.4 | 208 | 0–4 | 0.8* | 1.1 |
| Sentences to Dictation | 177 | 0–12 | 3.2 | 4.4 | 205 | 0–12 | 2.4 | 3.6 |

*Based on same scoring as in 1972. Revised scoring standards for these scales have been applied to 100 subjects to obtain percentiles that appear on the new score profile summary sheet.

tested in this battery. The first looks at intercorrelations between subtests representing each of nine functional dimensions, as revealed by inspection of an intercorrelation matrix. They are:

Overall severity of communicative impairment
Fluency of speech output
Auditory comprehension
Word finding
Repetition-recitation
Paraphasia
Reading
Writing
Visuospatial quantitative functions

As compared to the 1972 data, the intercorrelations within these clusters are higher. There are also a larger number of strong correlations between scores within the auditory comprehension cluster and those representing reading comprehension. These changes are probably due to the influence of the larger representation of very severe and moderately severe mixed aphasia, which tends to enhance

## SUBTEST SUMMARY PROFILE

NAME:                                     DATE OF EXAM:

| Category | PERCENTILES: | 0 | 10 | 20 | 30 | 40 | 50 | 60 | 70 | 80 | 90 | 100 |
|---|---|---|---|---|---|---|---|---|---|---|---|---|
| SEVERITY RATING | | | 0 | 1 | | | 2 | | | 3 | 4 | 5 |
| FLUENCY | ARTICULATION RATING | | 1 | 2 | 4 | 5 | 6 | | 7 | | | |
| | PHRASE LENGTH | | | 1 | 3 | 4 | 5 | 6 | 7 | | | |
| | MELODIC LINE | | 1 | 2 | 4 | | 6 | 7 | | | | |
| | VERBAL AGILITY | | 0 | 2 | 5 | 6 | 8 | 9 | 11 | 13 | 14 | |
| AUDITORY COMPREHENSION | WORD DISCRIMINATION | 0 | 15 | 25 | 37 | 46 | 53 | 60 | 64 | 67 | 70 | 72 |
| | BODY-PART IDENTIFICATION | 0 | 1 | 5 | 10 | 13 | 15 | 16 | 17 | 18 | | 20 |
| | COMMANDS | 0 | 3 | 4 | 6 | 8 | 10 | 11 | 13 | 14 | 15 | |
| | COMPLEX IDEATIONAL MATERIAL | | 0 | 2 | 3 | 4 | 5 | 6 | 8 | 9 | 11 | 12 |
| NAMING | RESPONSIVE NAMING | | | 0 | 1 | 5 | 10 | 15 | 20 | 24 | 27 | 30 |
| | CONFRONTATION NAMING | | 0 | 9 | 28 | 43 | 60 | 72 | 84 | 94 | 105 | 114 |
| | ANIMAL NAMING | | | 0 | 1 | 2 | 3 | 4 | 6 | | 9 | 23 |
| ORAL READING | WORD READING | | | 0 | 1 | 3 | 7 | 15 | 21 | 26 | 30 | |
| | ORAL SENTENCE READING | | | | 0 | 1 | 2 | 4 | 7 | 9 | | 10 |
| REPETITION | REPETITION OF WORDS | | 0 | 2 | 5 | 7 | 8 | | 9 | | 10 | |
| | HIGH-PROBABILITY | | | 0 | 1 | | 2 | 4 | 5 | 7 | 8 | |
| | LOW-PROBABILITY | | | | 0 | 1 | | | 2 | 4 | 6 | 8 |
| PARAPHASIA | NEOLOGISTIC | 40 | 16 | 9 | 4 | 2 | 1 | | 0 | | | |
| | LITERAL | 47 | 17 | 12 | 9 | 6 | 5 | 3 | 2 | 1 | 0 | |
| | VERBAL | 40 | 23 | 18 | 15 | 12 | 9 | 7 | 4 | 3 | 1 | 0 |
| | EXTENDED | 75 | 12 | 5 | 3 | 1 | 0 | | | | | |
| AUTOMATIC SPEECH | AUTOMATIZED SEQUENCES | | 0 | 1 | 2 | 3 | 4 | 6 | 7 | | 8 | |
| | RECITING | | | | 0 | 1 | | | | 2 | | |
| READING COMPREHENSION | SYMBOL DISCRIMINATION | 0 | 2 | 5 | 7 | 8 | 9 | | 10 | | | |
| | WORD RECOGNITION | 0 | 1 | 3 | 4 | 5 | 6 | 7 | | 8 | | |
| | COMPREHENSION OF ORAL SPELLING | | | | 0 | 1 | | 3 | 4 | 6 | 7 | 8 |
| | WORD-PICTURE MATCHING | | 0 | 1 | 4 | 6 | 8 | 9 | | 10 | | |
| | READING SENTENCES AND PARAGRAPHS | | 0 | 1 | 2 | 3 | 4 | 5 | 6 | 7 | 8 | 10 |
| WRITING | MECHANICS | 1 | | 2 | | 3 | | 4 | | 5 | | |
| | SERIAL WRITING | | 0 | 7 | 18 | 25 | 30 | 33 | 40 | 43 | 46 | 47 |
| | PRIMER-LEVEL DICTATION | | 0 | 1 | 4 | 6 | 9 | 11 | 13 | 14 | 15 | |
| | SPELLING TO DICTATION | | | | 0 | 1 | 2 | 3 | 5 | 7 | | 10 |
| | WRITTEN CONFRONTATION NAMING | | | 0 | 1 | 2 | 3 | 6 | 7 | 9 | | 10 |
| | SENTENCES TO DICTATION | | | | | 0 | 1 | 3 | | 6 | 8 | 12 |
| | NARRATIVE WRITING | | 0 | 1 | | | 2 | | | 3 | 4 | 5 |
| MUSIC | SINGING | | 0 | 1 | | 2 | | | | | | |
| | RHYTHM | | 0 | 1 | | | | 2 | | | | |
| SPATIAL AND COMPUTATIONAL | DRAWING TO COMMAND | 0 | 6 | 7 | 8 | 9 | 10 | 11 | 12 | | 13 | |
| | STICK MEMORY | 0 | 3 | 4 | 6 | 7 | 8 | 9 | 10 | 11 | 13 | 14 |
| | 3-D BLOCKS | | 0 | 2 | 4 | 5 | 6 | 7 | 8 | 9 | 10 | |
| | TOTAL FINGERS | 0 | 54 | 70 | 81 | 93 | 100 | 108 | 120 | 130 | 141 | 152 |
| | RIGHT-LEFT | 0 | 1 | 3 | 4 | 6 | 8 | 9 | 11 | 14 | 16 | |
| | MAP ORIENTATION | 0 | 2 | 5 | 6 | 9 | 11 | 13 | | 14 | | |
| | ARITHMETIC | | 0 | 2 | 4 | 8 | 11 | 14 | 17 | 21 | 27 | 32 |
| | CLOCK SETTING | 0 | 3 | 4 | 6 | | 8 | 9 | 10 | 12 | | |
| | | 0 | 10 | 20 | 30 | 40 | 50 | 60 | 70 | 80 | 90 | 100 |

**Fig. 1.** Subtest summary profile.

the relationships that vary as a function of severity.

The second approach is a series of factor analyses, carried out on several subsets of the measures in the battery, as well as on all of the measures taken together. Figuring in both approaches are the subtests of the supplementary nonlanguage tests (Chapter 6 of this manual), which tap visuospatial and quantitative abilities. The language tasks constitute 43 variables, and the nonlanguage tasks 23 more. The subjects were 252 aphasics, 10 of whom had received the aphasia battery only and 242 of whom received both the aphasia battery and the supplementary nonlanguage tests.

The clustering of the subtests is a clue to what may constitute significant psychologic components in the performance of aphasics. Any clusters that emerge must be interpreted with caution, however, because they are influenced both by the patient population and by the tests that happened to be chosen for the battery. This will become obvious in the review of the factor analyses in which the factorial structure varies considerably as a function of the subset of tasks included in the analysis. Moreover, once a pair of subtests is found to be correlated, the basis for the correlation may be either a common psychologic factor or the anatomic contiguity of the lesions affecting the two performances involved.

With respect to the effect of the sampling of patients, the emergence of independent performance factors depends on having a representation of patients with selective deficits of various kinds, some of which may be rare. Thus, in a population of patients with widespread damage of varying severity, there will be widespread impairment in all language modalities, varying in intensity from patient to patient. Correlational analysis of their test scores can be expected to yield high intercorrelations among all language performances, and factor analysis will yield an overwhelming first factor, produced by degrees of severity. If we look no further than the mathematical surface, we can accept this finding as indicating that aphasia is described adequately in terms of the impairment of a general language factor. Given the nature of lesions causing aphasia in an unselected population, the probability of a strong general severity factor is high. If such a population happened to include a single case of pure word deafness, an auditory receptive factor would still be rejected mathematically because a single case would have little influence on the correlations arising from the entire group. A quite different factorial structure can be expected in a sample of patients having highly selective deficits, corresponding to circumscribed focal lesions.

With these considerations in mind, we examine first the intercorrelations among measures that fall within the aforementioned functional clusters.

| Severity of Communication Impairment (correlations with severity rating scale) | | | |
|---|---|---|---|
| **High (rho more then .60)** | | **Low (rho less than .40)** | |
| Phrase-Length Rating | .62 | Articulatory Agility | .38 |
| Grammatical Form Rating | .65 | Word-Finding Rating | −.03 |
| Complex Comprehension | .61 | Neologistic Paraphasia | .29 |
| Responsive Naming | .78 | Literal Paraphasia | .07 |
| Confrontation Naming | .79 | Verbal Paraphasia | −.14 |
| Animal Naming | .69 | Extended Paraphasia | −.24 |
| Body-Part Naming | .74 | Mechanics of Writing | .32 |
| Word Reading | .64 | | |
| Oral Sentence Reading | .67 | | |
| Automatized Sequences | .65 | | |
| Serial Writing | .61 | | |
| Primer Dictation | .65 | | |
| Sentence Dictation | .69 | | |
| Narrative Writing | .71 | | |

Note that oral naming and complex auditory receptive tasks are most reflective of severity, as are the more complex reading comprehension and oral reading tasks. All of the writing tasks vary directly with severity. In contrast, the measures of motor facility in speech and writing are weakly correlated with severity, as are the counts of paraphasias of various types produced in oral production subtests. In contrast with the sensitivity of the naming tasks to severity, the word-finding rating scale is totally independent of this factor. As will become clear in the discussion of this rating scale (p. 33), the scale in fact was not designed to measure the absolute level of naming ability, but rather to reflect the balance between speech fluency and the availability of lexical words in running conversation.

| Fluency of Speech Output | | | | |
|---|---|---|---|---|
| | Verbal Agility | Melodic Line | Articulation Rating | Grammatical Form |
| Phrase Length | .68 | .90 | .64 | .93 |
| Verbal Agility | | .68 | .63 | .62 |
| Melodic Line Rating | | | .74 | .85 |
| Articulation Rating | | | | .59 |
| Grammatical Form | | | | |

| Auditory Comprehension | | | |
|---|---|---|---|
| | Body Parts | Commands | Complex Material |
| Word Discrimination | .83 | .80 | .69 |
| Body Parts | | .84 | .70 |
| Commands | | | .69 |

| Word Finding | | | | |
|---|---|---|---|---|
| | Visual Confrontation Naming | Oral Word Reading | Body-Part Naming | Animal Naming |
| Responsive Naming | .87 | .78 | .85 | .69 |
| Visual Confrontation Naming | | .87 | .90 | .70 |
| Oral Word Reading | | | .82 | .56 |
| Body-Part Naming* | | | | .71 |

*Body-Part Naming, which was introduced as an experimental subtest in the first edition, appears to be governed by exactly the same factors as Confrontation Naming, and it has therefore been eliminated as a separate subtest in the current edition.

| Recitation-Repetition | | | | | |
|---|---|---|---|---|---|
| | Verbal Agility | Reciting Verses | High-Probability Repetition | Low-Probability Repetition | Word Repetition |
| Automatic Sequences | .70 | .55 | .73 | .60 | .76 |
| Verbal Agility | | .49 | .65 | .58 | .75 |
| Reciting Verses | | | .60 | .59 | .54 |
| High-Probability Repetition | | | | .86 | .73 |
| Low-Probability Repetition | | | | | .60 |

| Paraphasia | | | |
|---|---|---|---|
| | Literal | Verbal | Extended Paraphasia (other) | Paraphasia Rating |
| Neologistic | .18 | .33 | .49 | −.55* |
| Literal | | .24 | .01 | −.49* |
| Verbal | | | −.24 | −.37* |
| Extended | | | | −.36* |

*Negative values in the last column are due to the fact that increasing counts in the variables of neologistic, literal, verbal, and extended paraphasia represent greater impairment, while higher ratings in the paraphasia rating scale represent fewer instances of paraphasia. The low intercorrelations in this subset of scores indicate either poor reliability or the fact that there are relatively few patients who have a similar propensity for various types of paraphasia.

| | | Reading | | | |
|---|---|---|---|---|---|
| | Oral Sentences | Symbol-Word Discrimination | Phonetic Word Recognition | Comprehension of Oral Spelling | Word-Picture Matching | Sentence and Paragraph Comprehension |
| Word Reading | .78 | .39 | .57 | .60 | .56 | .55 |
| Oral Sentences | | .31 | .51 | .63 | .41 | .54 |
| Symbol-Word Discrimination | | | .50 | .34 | .67 | .54 |
| Phonetic Word Recognition | | | | .52 | .66 | .55 |
| Comprehension of Oral Spelling | | | | | .41 | .49 |
| Word-Picture Matching | | | | | | .73 |

| | | Writing | | | |
|---|---|---|---|---|---|
| | Spelling to Dictation | Written Confrontation Naming | Narrative Writing | Serial Writing | Primer-Level Dictation | Sentences to Dictation |
| Writing Mechanics | .35 | .44 | .40 | .52 | .46 | .34 |
| Spelling to Dictation | | .85 | .75 | .64 | .64 | .77 |
| Written Naming | | | .77 | .75 | .71 | .71 |
| Narrative Writing | | | | .63 | .63 | .81 |
| Serial Writing | | | | | .80 | .57 |
| Primer Level Dictation | | | | | | .62 |

| | | Visuospatial-Quantitative | | | | |
|---|---|---|---|---|---|---|
| | Stick Design Memory | Total Fingers | Right-Left | Arithmetic | Clock Setting | 3-D Blocks | Map Orientation |
| Draw to Command | .60 | .48 | .37 | .56 | .59 | .61 | .52 |
| Stick Memory | | .42 | .37 | .58 | .63 | .63 | .43 |
| Total Fingers | | | .67 | .58 | .44 | .30 | .42 |
| Right-Left | | | | .62 | .43 | .41 | .37 |
| Arithmetic | | | | | .63 | .58 | .44 |
| Clock Setting | | | | | | .51 | .49 |
| 3-D Blocks | | | | | | | .43 |

## FACTOR ANALYSES

We report the findings in a series of factor analyses, using Promax rotation, which resulted in the cleanest separation of the variables in our battery. These factor analyses take into account not only the intercorrelations within the clusters defined a priori, which have just been summarized, but correlations that transcend these functional groupings. Data from 242 aphasics are included.

Table 3 presents a factor analysis based on inclusion of all the measures: i.e., the rating scales, the objective language subtests, and the nonverbal spatial-quantitative supplementary tests. Ten factors are isolated.

The first is most clearly related to the nonverbal spatial-quantitative tests, excluding those for finger identification; these subtests have loadings from .71 to .80 on Factor 1. Map orientation is less strongly represented than the others, with a loading of .45. Reading sentences and paragraphs is weakly represented (.41). No other language tasks are represented in this factor with loadings of .40 or greater. This factor appears to represent primarily a visuospatial-quantitative factor.

The second factor is a fluency factor, encompassing Melodic Line, Phrase Length, Articulatory Agility, and Grammatical Form ratings, and associated strongly with a tendency to "empty speech" on the rating scale for word-finding.

Factor 3, which is most typified by the Repetition subtests, Oral Sentence Reading, Recitation, and Verbal Agility, represents operations involving voluntary speech produc-

**Table 3.  Results of Factor Analysis Based on All Language and Nonlanguage Variables, Using All Subjects (only variables with loadings greater than .40 are listed)**

**Factor 1**
- Reading Sentences and Paragraphs .41
- Draw to Command .71
- Sticks from Memory .80
- Total Arithmetic .70
- Clocks .71
- 3-D Blocks .77
- Map Orientation .45

**Factor 2**
- Melodic Line Rating .84
- Phrase Length Rating .80
- Articulatory Agility Rating .52
- Grammatical Form Rating .85
- *Word-Finding Scale -.96
- Extended Paraphasia .51
- Serial Writing .47

**Factor 3**
- Verbal Agility .56
- Word-Reading .43
- Oral Sentences .86
- Repetition of Words .79
- Repetition (High-Probability) .58
- Repetition (Low-Probability) .47
- Automatized Sequences .67
- Reciting .49

**Factor 4**
- Auditory Comprehension (mean) .94
- Word Discrimination .77
- Body-Part Identification .68
- Commands .80
- Complex Ideation .69
- Symbol and Word Discrimination .43
- Word Recognition .45
- Finger Comprehension (Auditory) .52

**Factor 5**
- Comprehension of Oral Spelling .46
- Written Confrontation Naming .68
- Spelling to Dictation .90
- Sentences to Dictation .86
- Narrative Writing .82

**Factor 6**
- Verbal Paraphasia .59

**Factor 7**
- Oral Agility .83

**Factor 8**
- Finger-Name Comprehension .70
- Finger Total .41

**Factor 9**
- Visual Confrontation Naming .60
- Animal Naming .40
- Body-Part Naming .56
- Oral Word Reading .63
- Oral Sentence Reading .47
- Literal Paraphasia -.43
- Fingers Total .47

**Factor 10**
- Paraphasia Rating .81
- Literal Paraphasia .60

*Note that a negative trend on the word-finding rating scale reflects fluent, empty speech.

tion at the word level. It is characterized as a Repetition-Recitation factor.

Factor 4 sharply delineates the four auditory comprehension subtests, with loadings of .68 to .80. The mean of the auditory comprehension scores, as represented on the Rating Scale Profile, carries a loading of .94. Auditory comprehension of finger names appears with a loading of .52.

Factor 5 is determined almost exclusively by the writing tasks, from Spelling to Dictation through Narrative Writing (loadings from .68 to .90).

Verbal Paraphasia appears as a separate Factor 6 and Nonverbal Oral Agility as a separate Factor 7.

The Finger-Name Comprehension task, which was not significantly represented on the first (spatial-quantitative) factor, appears by itself as an eighth factor.

Factor 9 is highly selective for the four word-naming tasks—Visual Confrontation Naming, Animal Naming, Body-Part Naming, and Oral Word Reading, with minor representation of Oral Sentence Reading, Literal Paraphasia (negative loading), and Total Verbal Finger Identification score.

The tenth factor isolates two of the paraphasia scores: the Paraphasia rating scale and the Verbal Paraphasia count. The polarity of the loadings suggests that it be considered a "freedom from paraphasia" factor.

Summarizing this overall factor analysis, we have:

Factor 1—Spatial-Quantitative
Factor 2—Fluency
Factor 3—Repetition-Recitation
Factor 4—Auditory Comprehension
Factor 5—Writing
Factor 6—Verbal Paraphasia
Factor 7—Nonverbal Oral Agility
Factor 8—Finger Identification
Factor 9—Naming
Factor 10—Freedom from Paraphasia

In spite of the difference in the makeup of the population sample, these factors are remarkably similar to those derived in October, 1969, which consisted of Reading and Writing, Parietal Lobe Tests (here referred to as Spatial-Quantitative), Fluency-Repetition-Recitation, Auditory Comprehension, and

Paraphasia. The present factor analysis differs in deleting Reading as a separate factor, in separating fluency from the Repetition-Recitation factor, in identifying an important Naming factor, and in identifying minor factors for Verbal Oral Agility, Finger Recognition, and Freedom from Paraphasia.

A second factor analysis (Table 4), based only on the language measures and excluding the spatial-quantitative scales, yielded a factorial structure similar to the first. Beyond the deletion of the spatial-quantitative and finger recognition factors, reading now appears as an independent factor, and verbal paraphasia is no longer an independent factor, but appears as a component of a weak paraphasia factor. A summary of the factors from the second analysis follows:

|  |  | Eigenvalue |
|---|---|---|
| Factor 1 | Auditory Comprehension | 9.6 |
| Factor 2 | Fluency | 6.2 |
| Factor 3 | Repetition-Recitation | 12.0 |
| Factor 4 | Writing | 11.5 |
| Factor 5 | Oral Agility (nonverbal) | 4.8 |
| Factor 6 | Reading | 10.9 |
| Factor 7 | Paraphasia | 2.5 |

A rigorous computation of the amount of variance accounted for by each factor is not possible with Promax rotation, since there is some correlation between factors. Since these eigenvalues are in direct proportion to the variance for each factor, however, we can conclude that the Auditory Comprehension, Repetition-Recitation, Reading, and Writing factors are of roughly equal importance and the Fluency factor somewhat less so; the Paraphasia factor is relatively minor.

A third factor analysis was compiled, deleting the variables from the Rating Scale Profile that contain most of the measures relating to Fluency. The result is displayed in Table 5, in which there are four factors of approximately equivalent importance and one minor factor. Factor 1 is a composite of basic comprehension, naming, and reading measures, on which the reading tasks have the highest loadings. It is probably best characterized as a Reading factor.

In Factor 2, the Recitation-Repetition cluster reappears, again with significant representation of the basic naming measures (Visual Confrontation and Body-Part Naming). In this sense, the factor may be taken as re-

**Table 4. Factor Analysis of Language Measures**

| Factor: 1 | 2 | 3 | 4 | 5 | 6 | 7 |
|---|---|---|---|---|---|---|
| Word-Finding Rating −.89 | Melodic Line Rating .88 | Paraphasia Severity Rating .48 | Comprehension of Oral Spelling .52 | Oral Agility .93 | Word Discrimination .40 | Paraphasia Severity Rating .99 |
| Auditory Comprehension .84 | Phrase Length Rating .87 | Verbal Agility .65 | Serial Writing .48 | Mechanics of Writing .44 | Confrontation Naming .50 | Literal Paraphasia .48 |
| Word Discrimination .63 | Articulatory Agility Rating .87 | Responsive Naming .44 | Primer-Level Dictation .47 | | Oral Word Reading .51 | Verbal Paraphasia .44 |
| Body-Part Identification .65 | Grammatical Form Rating .92 | Confrontation Naming .45 | Written Naming .75 | | Symbol and Word Discrimination .53 | |
| Commands .78 | Extended Paraphasia .48 | Body-Part Naming .50 | Spelling to Dictation .83 | | Word Recognition .47 | |
| Complex Ideational Material .68 | | Oral Word Reading .56 | Sentences to Dictation .78 | | Word-Picture Matching .83 | |
| | | Repetition of Words 1.00 | Narrative Writing .79 | | Reading Sentences and Paragraphs .72 | |
| | | Repetition (High-Probability) .79 | | | Serial Writing .48 | |
| | | Repetition (Low-Probability) .60 | | | | |
| | | Neologisms − .61 | | | | |
| | | Automatized Sequences .75 | | | | |
| | | Recitation .54 | | | | |

**Table 5.  Factor Analysis of Language Variables, Excluding Rating Scale Measures**

| Factor: 1 | | 2 | | 3 | | 4 | | 5 | |
|---|---|---|---|---|---|---|---|---|---|
| Word Discrimination | .52 | Verbal Agility | .81 | Comprehension of Oral Spelling | .40 | Oral Agility | .42 | Word Discrimination | .47 |
| Confrontation Naming | .52 | Responsive Naming | .51 | Writing Mechanics | .45 | Singing | .40 | Body-Part Identification | .57 |
| Body-Part Naming | .47 | Confrontation Naming | .52 | Serial Writing | .46 | Rhythm | .48 | Commands | .66 |
| Word Reading | .60 | Body-Part Naming | .52 | Primer-Level Dictation | .42 | | | Complex Ideational Material | .55 |
| Extended Paraphasia | −.42 | Oral Sentence Reading | .41 | Written Naming | .76 | | | Comprehension of Oral Spelling | .44 |
| Symbol and Word Discrimination | .57 | Repetition of Words | .99 | Spelling to Dictation | .78 | | | | |
| Word Recognition | .50 | Repetition (High-Probability) | .76 | Sentences to Dictation | .77 | | | | |
| Word-Picture Matching | .83 | Repetition (Low-Probability) | .60 | Narrative Writing | .88 | | | | |
| Reading Sentences and Paragraphs | .66 | Automatized Sequences | .85 | | | | | | |
| Serial Writing | .40 | Reciting | .48 | | | | | | |

flecting the capacity for voluntary speech production.

Factor 3 is a clearcut Writing factor, and Factor 5 is an Auditory Comprehension factor. A new minor factor, Factor 4, has loadings in the .40s for Oral Agility, Singing, and Rhythm.

Thus, removal of the measures of fluency also results in redistribution of the factorial membership of other variables. Naming now appears equally associated with the Reading and Recitation-Repetition factors, while Paraphasia is unrepresented.

A fourth factor analysis (Table 6) was computed on 23 variables of the Aphasia test that had unskewed, normal distributions. The outcome yielded two factors. Factor 1 is now a composite of both auditory and written receptive tasks, with elementary writing at the one-word level. Factor 2 is a Speech Production Factor, most heavily representing Repetition and Verbal Agility, but with important loadings for the naming tasks.

A final factor analysis was carried out, using only 41 subjects who had been selected as prototypical Broca's (9), Wernicke's (12), conduction (10), and anomic (10) aphasics, and the variables with loadings of over .40 on the eight factors are displayed in Table 7. The factors appear to be identifiable under the following labels:

| | | Eigenvalue |
|---|---|---|
| 1. | Repetition | 8.7 |
| 2. | Auditory Comprehension | 10.1 |
| 3. | Writing | 8.0 |
| 4. | Fluency | 6.2 |
| 5. | Singing | 2.5 |
| 6. | Naming | 10.2 |
| 7. | Uninterpretable | 6.8 |
| 8. | Verbal Paraphasia | 2.9 |

Again, the eigenvalues are provided as an approximate indication of the relative significance of the factors in accounting for the total variance.

Since this factor analysis differed from the second only in the fact that here patients were selected for prototypicality as representatives of four diagnostic types, the differences in the factorial structure can be attributed to the characteristics of the population. The main differences lie in the disappearance of a separate reading factor and in the heightened prominence of repetition as the major component of Factor 1. Auditory Comprehension, Writing, Fluency, and Naming retain their identity as separable factors.

The added prominence of repetition as a key variable may be attributed to the relatively large representation of conduction aphasics in this selected sample. This interpretation is supported by the fact of the strong, opposite loading of literal paraphasia, which is to be expected from the fact that conduction aphasics show an unusual impairment of repetition,

**Table 6. Factor Analysis of Normally Distributed Language Variables**

| Factor: 1 | | 2 | |
|---|---|---|---|
| Word Discrimination | .91 | Verbal Agility | .84 |
| Body-Part Identification | .77 | Responsive Naming | .59 |
| Commands | .73 | Confrontation Naming | .66 |
| Complex Ideational Material | .54 | Body-Part Naming | .62 |
| Responsive Naming | .41 | Word Reading | .62 |
| Animal Naming | .43 | Oral Sentence Reading | .62 |
| Symbol Discrimination | .78 | Repetition of Words | .90 |
| Word Recognition | .65 | Repetition (High-Probability) | .84 |
| Comprehensive Oral Spelling | .40 | Automatized Sequences | .91 |
| Word-Picture Matching | .92 | Comprehension of Oral Spelling | .40 |
| Reading Sentences and Paragraphs | .73 | | |
| Serial Writing | .64 | | |
| Primer-Level Dictation | .71 | | |
| Written Naming | .57 | | |

along with an unusually great number of literal paraphasias in naming tasks.

## DISCRIMINANT ANALYSIS

In our view, the allocation of an aphasic patient's pattern of deficits to one of the named syndromes is based on a number of criteria that, at best, are imperfectly reduced to measurable dimensions and involve some features that cannot be defined at all in quantitative terms. In addition, the experienced clinician assigns heavy weighting to particular features that may appear in classic and florid form in a particular case. For example, impairments in auditory comprehension will be weighted by the clinician according to the patient's speed and apparent assurance in indicating his comprehension of words, as well as according to signs that fatigue, confusability, or perseveration are contaminating a comprehension score. Similarly, judgments applied to the quality of articulatory difficulty of paraphasias, and of grammatical usage, will cause the experienced clinician to make a diagnostic allocation that is not totally in accord with a quantitative definition of a syndrome. Furthermore, as we discuss elsewhere (p. 74), a minority of cases are unambiguous exemplars of a single syndrome.

With these cautions in mind, we undertook to provide the user of this test with an improved basis for deriving diagnostic classifications from test score configurations, through the outcome of a discriminant analysis. This was possible only for the four major categories of Broca's, Wernicke's, anomic, and conduction aphasia, because insufficient instances (approximately ten) of each of other diagnostic types could be identified in our files. The procedure for selecting cases began with a printout of all subjects who had been assigned unequivocally to a particular category. These were then reviewed by one of us to select as close as possible to ten prototypical cases, on the basis of the clinical narrative description by the neurologist, the location of the lesion site, and the test scores. The number of prototypical cases for each category was as follows:

| | |
|---|---|
| Broca's aphasia | 9 |
| Wernicke's aphasia | 14 |
| Conduction aphasia | 10 |
| Anomic aphasia | 10 |

Ten variables were selected on the a priori presumption that they would provide the most useful data for discriminating the foregoing groups. They were:

Verbal Agility Score
Body-Part Identification
Repetition of High-Probability Sentences
Paraphasia Rating
Word-Finding Rating
Grammatical Form Rating
Phrase-Length Rating
Automatized Sequences
Articulatory Agility Rating
Verbal Paraphasia Count

The most effective separation of subjects

**Table 7. Factor Analysis of Language Variables, Using Data from 41 Prototypical Cases of Four Diagnostic Subgroups**

| Factor: 1 | 2 | 3 | 4 | 5 | 6 | 7 | 8 |
|---|---|---|---|---|---|---|---|
| Phrase Length Rating .44 | Paraphasia Severity Rating .43 | Body-Part Naming .53 | Melodic Line Rating .93 | Word Recognition .56 | Paraphasia Severity Rating .55 | Auditory Comprehension (mean) .43 | Verbal Paraphasia .80 |
| Paraphasia Severity Rating .73 | Auditory Comprehension (mean) .96 | Confrontation Naming .45 | Phrase Length Rating .95 | Singing .73 | Auditory Comprehension Rating .46 | Verbal Agility .47 | Comprehension of Oral Spelling .49 |
| Verbal Agility .79 | Word Discrimination .92 | Oral Sentence Reading .60 | Articulation Rating .78 | | Word Discrimination .55 | Word Discrimination .49 | |
| Responsive Naming .64 | Body-Part Identification .87 | Repetition (High-Probability) .45 | Grammatical Form Rating .88 | | Body-Part Identification .47 | Body-Part Identification .53 | |
| Confrontation Naming .63 | Commands .85 | Repetition (Low-Probability) .47 | Word-Finding Rating −.80 | | Responsive Naming .69 | Commands .43 | |
| Repetition of Words .82 | Complex Ideational Material .86 | Verbal Paraphasia .42 | Verbal Agility .68 | | Confrontation Naming .86 | Confrontation Naming .56 | |
| Repetition (High-Probability) .83 | Responsive Naming .75 | Comprehension of Oral Spelling .63 | Automatized Sequences .55 | | Animal Naming .79 | Body-Part Naming .63 | |
| Repetition (Low-Probability) .80 | Animal Naming .48 | Mechanics of Writing .47 | Reciting .43 | | Body-Part Naming .77 | Word Reading .44 | |
| Neologisms −.44 | Confrontation Naming .48 | Serial Writing .65 | | | Word Reading .86 | Repetition of Words .64 | |
| Literal Paraphasia −.72 | Body-Part Naming .55 | Primer-Level Dictation .65 | | | Oral Sentences .76 | Repetition (High-Probability) .45 | |
| Automatized Sequences .75 | Word Reading .41 | Written Naming .83 | | | Repetition of Words .51 | Neologisms −.46 | |
| Reciting .70 | Oral Sentences .41 | Spelling to Dictation .65 | | | Repetition (High-Probability) .41 | Extended Paraphasia −.56 | |
| Comprehension of Oral Spelling .44 | Repetition (High-Probability) .48 | Sentences to Dictation .87 | | | Repetition (Low Probability) .41 | Automatized Sequences .52 | |
| | Repetition (Low-Probability) .51 | Narrative Writing .91 | | | Neologisms −.71 | Word Recognition .72 | |
| | Extended Paraphasia −.67 | | | | Extended Paraphasia −.45 | Word-Picture Matching .48 | |
| | Reciting .46 | | | | Automatized Sequences .48 | Serial Writing .51 | |
| | Symbol and Word Discrimination .53 | | | | Symbol and Word Discrimination .55 | Primer-Level Dictation .64 | |
| | Word Recognition .50 | | | | Word Recognition .62 | Rhythm .75 | |
| | Comprehension of Oral Spelling .69 | | | | Comprehension of Oral Spelling .43 | | |
| | | | | | Word-Picture Matching .56 | | |
| | | | | | Reading Sentences and Paragraphs .65 | | |
| | | | | | Serial Writing .69 | | |
| | | | | | Primer Dictation .51 | | |
| | | | | | Written Naming .46 | | |

was based on entering five of these variables into the discriminant analysis. These were:

Body-Part Identification
Repetition of High-Probability Sentences
Verbal Paraphasia
Articulatory Agility Rating
Automatized Sequences

This set of variables yielded the following classification matrix, in which the column "Other" represents subjects who did not attain a probability of .70 or more for assignment to a particular diagnosis. There are 41 subjects in this analysis, because 2 of the Wernicke's aphasics had incomplete data.

| | Broca | Wernicke | Predicted: Conduction | Anomic | Other |
|---|---|---|---|---|---|
| Actual: | | | | | |
| Broca | 9 | 0 | 0 | 0 | 0 |
| Wernicke | 0 | 11 | 0 | 0 | 1 |
| Conduction | 0 | 0 | 10 | 0 | 0 |
| Anomic | 0 | 0 | 0 | 10 | 0 |

(no misclassifications; one "other")

A second discriminant analysis used 43 subjects and the following 6 variables:

Body-Part Identification
Repetition of High-Probability Sentences
Paraphasia Rating
Word-Finding Rating
Phrase-Length Rating
Verbal Paraphasia

This analysis resulted in one misclassification of an Anomic and a Wernicke's aphasic, and one failure to reach .70 probability in the case of one patient diagnosed as a Wernicke's aphasic.

The discriminant analyses just described have not been cross validated. It is possible to obtain indices for comparing the relative likelihood of assignment to any of the four diagnostic categories by applying the following weighting formulas to any subject's scores:

All test score values in the formulas are *raw scores* (not percentiles).

For Group 1 (Broca's aphasia): [(1.13 × Body-Part Identification) + (0.1 × High-Probability Repetition) + (3.0 × Articulation Rating) + (0.1 × Automatized Sequences) + (0.1 × Verbal Paraphasia Count) − 17.8]

For Group 2 (Wernicke's aphasia): [(0.6 × Body-Part Identification) − (1.3 × High-Probability Repetition) + (6.2 × Articulation Rating) + (1.0 × Automatized Sequences) + (0.1 × Verbal Paraphasia) − 26.7]

For Group 3 (Conduction aphasia): [(1.1 × Body-Part Identification) + (1.6 × High-Probability Repetition) + (5.8 × Articulation Rating) − (0.2 × Automatized Sequences) − 37.2]

For Group 4 (Anomic aphasia): [(1.2 × Body-Part Identification) − (1.4 × High-Probability Repetition) + (5.7 × Articulation Rating) + (0.6 × Automatized Sequences) + (0.2 × Verbal Paraphasia) − 31.1]

The formula that yields the highest value represents the most likely diagnostic assignment. Since transcortical aphasics and global aphasics were not included in the discriminant analysis, applying these formulas to global aphasics or to patients with relatively high repetition scores will give spurious results. It is clear that one of the formulas will give a highest value for any patient, so this method should be used with selected patients only. When applied to 41 selected prototypical cases, 37 were correctly classified. It must be stressed, too, that in the absence of cross validation, one cannot expect such a high "hit" rate on new cases.

There is a second and more flexible way of using the outcome of the discriminant analysis, which is to plot the location of a set of scores in a two-dimensional space defined by the two discriminant functions. The standardized discriminant function coefficients are as follows:

| | Function 1 | Function 2 |
|---|---|---|
| Body-Part Identification | 0.39 | −0.37 |
| High-Probability Repetition | 1.05 | 0.44 |
| Articulation Rating | −0.36 | 0.72 |
| Automatized Sequences | −0.64 | 0.11 |
| Verbal Paraphasias | −0.21 | −0.20 |

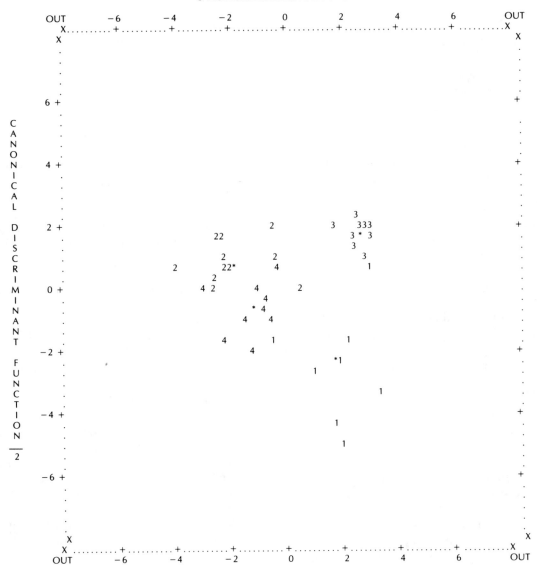

ALL-GROUPS SCATTERPLOT – * INDICATES A GROUP CENTROID

CANONICAL DISCRIMINANT FUNCTION 1

**Fig. 2.** Scatter plot of distribution of 37 correctly classified prototypical cases of Broca's (1), Wernicke's (2), conduction (3), and anomic aphasics (4) in terms of two discriminant functions.

**Table 8.  Means, Standard Deviations, Ranges, and Cutoff Scores for Normal Performance on the BDAE**

| Subtest | Mean | SD | Range | Suggested Cutoff Score | Exceptions |
|---|---|---|---|---|---|
| Word Discrimination | 71.8 | .6 | 67–72 | 67 | |
| Body-Part Identification | 19.7 | .5 | 18–20 | 18 | |
| Commands | 14.9 | .4 | 13–15 | 13 | |
| Complex Ideational Material | 11.2 | 1.1 | 7–12 | 8 | below grade 9 |
| Oral Agility: | | | | | |
| Nonverbal Agility | 10.4 | 1.5 | 6–12 | 9 | 60 years or over |
| Verbal Agility | 13.7 | .6 | 11–14 | 11 | |
| Automatized Sequences | 7.9 | .3 | 6–8 | 6 | |
| Reciting | 1.9 | .3 | 0–2 | 1* | |
| Singing | 1.8 | .5 | 0–2 | 0 | |
| Rhythm | 1.8 | .5 | 0–2 | 0 | |
| Repetition of Words | 9.9 | .3 | 9–10 | 9 | |
| Repeating Phrases: | | | | | |
| High Probability | 7.9 | .4 | 6–8 | 6 | |
| Low Probability | 7.7 | .6 | 5–8 | 6* | |
| Responsive Naming | 29.9 | .5 | 27–30 | 27 | |
| Body-Part Naming† | 29.4 | 1.2 | 24–30 | 24 | |
| Animal Naming | 22.5 | 6.8 | 9–41 | 12 | 60 years or over |
| Oral Sentence Reading | 9.9 | .4 | 8–10 | 8 | |
| Word Recognition | 7.9 | .3 | 6–8 | 6 | |
| Comprehension of Oral Spelling | 7.7 | .7 | 4–8 | 6* | |
| Reading Sentences and Paragraphs | 9.5 | .8 | 7–10 | 7 | |
| Spelling to Dictation | 8.9 | 1.2 | 4–10 | 6* | |
| Written Confrontation Naming | 9.7 | .6 | 7–10 | 7 | |
| Narrative Writing† | 3.7 | .5 | 2–4 | 2 | |
| Sentences Written to Dictation | 11.9 | .4 | 10–12 | 10 | |

*Indicates cutoff based on two standard deviations below the mean.
†Applies to 1972 version of BDAE.

It appears that Function 1 is determined most heavily by repetition; Function 2, by articulation. In order to determine the score of any individual on these two functions, the following two formulas are computed:

Function 1 = [(0.14) + (0.11 × Body-Part Identification) + (0.63 × High-Probability Repetition) − (0.34 × Articulation Rating) − (0.26 × Automatic Sequences) − (0.03 × Verbal Paraphasia)]

Function 2 = [(−3.5) + (0.27 × High-Probability Repetition) + (0.69 × Articulation Rating) + (0.05 × Automatized Sequences) + (0.03 × Verbal Paraphasia) − (0.10 × Body-Part Identification)]

Group centroids derived from these formulas are as follows:

|  | Function 1 | Function 2 |
|---|---|---|
| Broca (Group 1) | 1.58 | −2.29 |
| Wernicke (Group 2) | −1.97 | 0.80 |
| Conduction (Group 3) | 2.33 | 1.79 |
| Anomic (Group 4) | −1.39 | −0.70 |

Figure 2 shows the distribution of cases, identified by their group number on a scatter plot, in which Function 1 is the abscissa and Function 2 the ordinate. The centroids for the four groups appear as asterisks. This scatter plot shows that anomic and Wernicke's aphasics may be misclassified for each other in terms of the five variables from which the discriminant is derived.

This scatter plot may prove valuable for other types of patients. Its major advantage is that patients whose symptoms are on the boundary of two diagnostic types may be seen to fall in a boundary location.

PERFORMANCE OF NORMAL SUBJECTS. The Boston Diagnostic Aphasia Examination was administered to 147 neurologically normal English-speaking men, ranging in age from 25 to 85 years and in education from less than 8 grades through college (Borod, Goodglass, and Kaplan, 1980). Seven of the subtests were deleted from this norming procedure, on the presumption that no failures should be anticipated from nonaphasic adults. The deleted subtests were Oral Word Reading, Visual Confrontation Naming, Symbol and Word Discrimination, Word-Picture Matching, Mechanics of Writing, Serial Writing, and Primer-Level Dictation. The results of this data collection are summarized in Table 8. With few exceptions, the mean is within a fraction of a point of the maximum possible score, although the lowest scores (reflected in the column marked "Range") indicate that a few individuals fell short of the maximum raw score by as much as five or six points on four subtests. Low scorers were invariably in the group of subjects over 60 years of age with fewer than 9 years of schooling. A suggested cutoff score is given, determined in most cases by the lowest scoring normal, but in instances in which a single outlier produced a deviantly low score, the suggested cutoff score is two standard deviations below the mean.

# CHAPTER 4

# Test Procedures and Rationale: Manual for the Boston Diagnostic Aphasia Test

This chapter constitutes an administration manual, supplementing the instructions in the test booklet, where the latter are not self explanatory.

Prior to administration of the test, the vital background data necessary to orient the clinician to the educational, vocational, and medical history of the patient should be recorded on the face sheet of the test booklet.

## CONVERSATIONAL AND EXPOSITORY SPEECH

This section of the test booklet is designed to determine the level and quality of the patient's speech and comprehension under conditions of open-ended conversation and free narrative. If possible, it should be tape-recorded. Playback of the tape will greatly facilitate completing the Rating Scale Profile of Speech Characteristics. This scale covers those features that are most resistant to quantification, and will supplement the more objective scores obtained from the rest of the examination.

Items "a" through "g" provide an inventory of common expressions available as responses in conversational give-and-take. They include the ability to reply appropriately to a greeting, to answer with "yes" or "no," to say "I think so," "I don't know," "I hope so," or their equivalents. The questions in the test booklet, sug-

gested to elicit these expressions, need not be followed verbatim, particularly if the patient's level of speech is obviously above that demanded to answer them. Items "f" and "g" ask for name and address and should always be included, since severely anomic patients may fail with these specific information-giving items in spite of being deceptively fluent in the opening small talk.

Item "h" places more demand on the patient for talking freely without a specific stimulus. Avoid asking "yes-no" questions in encouraging the patient to elaborate, since these merely put a damper on conversation. Whenever possible, conversation should be continued for about 10 minutes. A sample of this length is likely to give the patient an opportunity to demonstrate his speech fluency, even though his opening conversation may be rather halting. Many milder anomic patients, however, begin to falter and make errors in speech after a beginning in which no speech difficulty is apparent for several minutes. The degree of fluency should be judged in terms of the subject's best performance.

The conversation is terminated at the discretion of the examiner, who then presents item "i"—a picture situation (the Cookie Theft) with instructions to "Tell all about what you see going on in this picture." If a tape recording is being made to facilitate rating, it should be continued through the picture description. It will be noted that the quality of the speech pattern often changes drastically in the shift from free conversation to picture description. The reason is that some anomic patients have the knack of moving about from one available expression to another in free conversation, while completely avoiding the words that they sense as a source of trouble. The vocabulary constraints of the picture bring out the word-finding difficulty more sharply.

### Use of Rating Scale Profile of Speech Characteristics, Severity Rating, and Subtest Summary Profile

Six features of speech production, which are not satisfactorily measured by objective scores, are to be rated during or immediately after concluding the conversational and expository speech interview (Figure 3). If a tape recording has been made, rating may be deferred and done during a playback of the recording, which is preferable to rating the live interview. Rating is done more reliably when the rater can concentrate on listening for the critical features that may escape him when he is busy interviewing.

The six features are: melodic line, phrase length, articulatory agility, grammatical form (variety of grammatical constructions), paraphasia in running speech, and word finding. Two additional scales, one for repetition and one for auditory comprehension, are based on a conversion of the objective test scores. Seven of the ratings are on a seven-point scale, on which "7" stands for minimum abnormality and "1" stands for maximum abnormality. The scale for word-finding ability is deviant at both extremes, as explained in the following.

The severity rating is a scale of capacity for oral communication ranging from "0" for "no communication possible" to "5" for "no perceptible handicap." The Profile of Speech Characteristics must be interpreted in the light of the severity rating. The steps of the severity rating are defined on the scale record form (Figure 3).

The Subtest Summary Profile (Figure 1), also included in the test booklet, provides raw scores for each subtest of the Boston Diagnostic Aphasia Examination, as well as the ratings assigned for severity, articulation, phrase length, and melodic line. The position of the raw score on its horizontal line may be read off as a percentile from the scale at the top and bottom of the page. The percentile score gives the standing of the corresponding raw score in terms of the percentage of the population that had a lower score. Thus, the median score is at the fiftieth percentile. This permits a direct comparison of performance level on tests whose raw scores may have totally disparate ranges.

### Rationale and Rules for Assigning Profile Ratings

The rules for assigning profile ratings may appear somewhat arbitrary at some points, particularly in relation to the Melodic Line, Phrase-Length, and Paraphasia ratings. The rules have been designed to allow the scales to discriminate maximally between aphasics of differing diagnostic types who have dramatically different clinical features.

MELODIC LINE. This term refers to the intonational pattern that normally encompasses the entire sentence and that includes rise in pitch, volume, and duration on stressed words, slight raising of pitch, which indicates a syntactic juncture where there is more to follow, and the final intonation, which signals a question, declarative, or command. In the most severely dysrhythmic and amelodic speech production, there may be no intonational link between words or even between syllables; words are spoken as though being enumerated rather than grouped syntactically. At the intermediate level "4," the normal melodic line may extend to three- or four-word expressions of a stereotyped nature, such as "I can't say it." Patients whose sentences or uninterrupted utterances *never* exceed four words in length cannot receive a rating of more than "4." The reason for this rule is that the Melodic Line Rating is most valuable as an index of the character of extended utterances. If short or stereotyped utterances were to be given a rating of normal melodic line, this scale would no longer distinguish between those patients who can impose appropriate intonation on complex sentences from those

## APHASIA SEVERITY RATING SCALE

0.  No usable speech or auditory comprehension.

1.  All communication is through fragmentary expression; great need for inference, questioning, and guessing by the listener. The range of information that can be exchanged is limited, and the listener carries the burden of communication.

2.  Conversation about familiar subjects is possible with help from the listener. There are frequent failures to convey the idea, but patient shares the burden of communication with the examiner.

3.  The patient can discuss almost all everyday problems with little or no assistance. Reduction of speech and/or comprehension, however, makes conversation about certain material difficult or impossible.

4.  Some obvious loss of fluency in speech or facility of comprehension, without significant limitation on ideas expressed or form of expression.

5.  Minimal discernible speech handicaps; patient may have subjective difficulties that are not apparent to listener.

## RATING SCALE PROFILE OF SPEECH CHARACTERISTICS

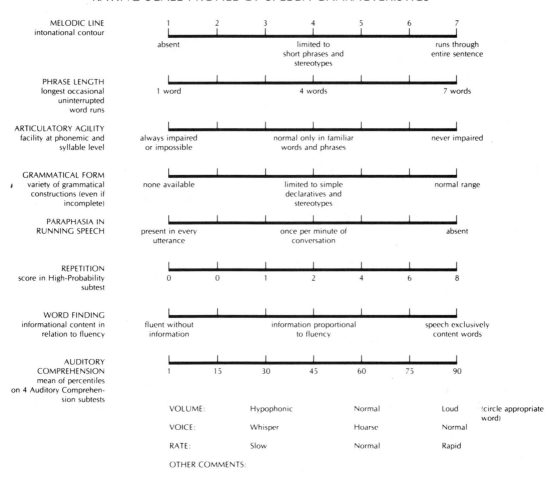

**Fig. 3.** Aphasia severity rating scale and rating scale profile of speech characteristics.

who can produce only short sentences with appropriate prosody.

PHRASE LENGTH. This quality is measured by the length of uninterrupted runs of words, set off at either end by a pause or sentence boundary. The numeric steps of the scale represent the longest number of words per run that occurs at least once in about 10 starts by the patient. Thus, this rating is *not* the average length of uninterrupted word groupings, but the longest grouping that may be expected occasionally. If, for example, in 30 utterances, 3 contain 6 or more words without a break, the scale rating is "6," even if one of the occasions extended to 10 words and even though the majority of the utterances are aborted after 3 to 4 words. The criterion of 1 in 10 is given as a guide for estimation by the rater. The reason for this rule is that patients who are judged clinically to have a fluent speech pattern may have many utterances that are aborted after a few words because of word-finding problems. Thus, the feature of fluency in speech output is best indexed by the occasional longest connected utterances, rather than by the average length. For the degree of precision expected in this rating, it is sufficient to listen to the recorded sample with particular attention to the occasional longest uninterrupted runs.

ARTICULATION RATING. The ease with which the patient articulates phonemic sequences constitutes articulatory agility. The examiner should listen for any awkwardness, explosive word onset, groping for initial sounds, simplification of consonant blends or sound substitutions *due to articulatory difficulty.* If every word is produced with normal ease, the patient receives a maximum score here. Literal paraphasia, i.e., sound transpositions or contaminations in a setting of facile articulation, does not constitute a loss of articulatory agility for purposes of this rating. The rating is based on the prevalence, as much as the severity, of impaired articulation. A rating of "1" indicates articulatory difficulty in every utterance. The middle score of "4" indicates that articulation is normal only in brief, relatively overlearned expressions. Two interpolated steps are provided between the midpoint and each extreme.

GRAMMATICAL FORM. This encompasses the continuum from "agrammatic" or one-word-sentence speech to a normal variety of grammatical forms. At severe levels, isolated nouns predominate, and one rarely hears syntactic combinations beyond verb plus object. The verb is usually unmarked with respect to tense. At moderate levels, the patient constructs simple declarative sentences in the present or past tense, but does not deviate from the "subject-verb-object" sequence and never starts a sentence with a subordinate clause. At normal levels, one hears longer sentences with subordinate clauses, conditionals, future tenses, and passive constructions. Many patients who use a variety of grammatical forms may leave sentences incomplete because of word-finding difficulty; in addition, their grammar may be flawed by their semantic misuse of words (paraphasia). Paraphasic errors and aborted sentences are compatible with normal ratings for "variety of grammatical forms."

PARAPHASIA IN RUNNING SPEECH. The focus here is not on paraphasic substitutions of individual nouns in one-word responses as seen in aphasics of many types, but rather on the substitutions or insertions of semantically erroneous words in running conversation, which is diagnostically significant. For this scale, not only semantic errors but partially or completely neologistic errors are noted, and the score depends chiefly on the prevalence of such errors. The maximum abnormality of "1" implies paraphasia included in every utterance; the minimum of "7" implies complete absence of such errors. The midpoint of "4" represents an average of a paraphasic error in approximately each minute of conversation.

*This scale does not apply to patients whose Phrase-Length Rating is 3 or less.* Paraphasias produced by these patients rarely have significance for diagnostic distinctions. It may be left blank or assigned an arbitrary rating of "7" for patients who cannot produce any running speech. The following are *not* considered paraphasic: Recurring use of a small repertory of words or syllables; continuous output of syllables without clear segmentation into word-like units, especially when they involve a limited repertory of consonant-vowel combinations.

REPETITION. Unlike the preceding variables on this profile chart, repetition can be measured reasonably well by an objective test, in this case, the score on Repetition of High-Probability Phrases. The only purpose of inserting this variable in the profile is that it adds a diagnostically distinctive feature that aids in identifying conduction aphasics (repetition worse than comprehension) and transcortical aphasics (repetition remarkably well preserved). The seven scale positions represent the scores of the first, fifteenth, thirtieth, forty-fifth, sixtieth, seventy-fifth and ninetieth percentiles.

Conversions on this subtest, indicated in the test booklet, are as follows:

| Scale Rating: | 1 | 2 | 3 | 4 | 5 | 6 | 7 |
|---|---|---|---|---|---|---|---|
| Percentile: | 1 | 15 | 30 | 45 | 60 | 75 | 90 |
| Raw Score: | 0 | 0 | 1 | 2 | 4 | 6 | 8 |

WORD FINDING. The patient's capacity to evoke needed concept names is reflected in the informational content of his speech; however, the rating is made with respect to the level of fluency. In a quantitative sense, it reflects the proportion of substantives and specific action-words to the number of low-information words, i.e., grammatical connectives, pronouns, auxiliary verbs, indefinite words such as "something" and other compounds of "thing," "place," "body." A rating of "7" stands for speech consisting almost exclusively of substantives and picturable actions. The relative dearth of low-information words is usually reflected in short or agrammatic sentence forms, a characteristic that tends to correlate with this scale. The middle rating of "4" means that the examiner estimates the proportion of specific nouns and verbs to be just appropriate to the fluency level. A rating of "1" indicates fluent speech in which virtually no specific nouns or verbs occur. Such speech, which we call "empty speech," is usually grammatically organized, but vague and circumlocutory, with the same expressions recurring frequently.

Unlike the other scales, this one does not represent normal performance at step "7" and most deviant at step "1." In fact, the patient rated "7" may have great difficulty in naming. The rating of "7" indicates only that the naming function is so much better preserved than grammatical fluency that output consists almost entirely of content-words.

AUDITORY COMPREHENSION. As in the case of repetition, and unlike the other variables on this profile chart, auditory comprehension can be adequately measured by objective test scores. It, too, has been included on the chart because of its contribution to the distinctive appearance of profiles of the various diagnostic groups of aphasics. The entry on this scale is based on the mean percentile score of the four auditory comprehension subtests, as plotted on the Subtest Summary Profile.

## Reliability of the Ratings

In the development of the Profile of Speech Characteristics, judgments were made independently by three raters, listening to the tape-recorded conversation. The ratings used were the mean of the three judges' ratings for each scale. In order to assess the reliability of the individual judges' ratings, we computed Pearson product moment correlations, across 99 subjects, between the two most disparate ratings on each scale, this being the most stringent approach possible. The correlation coefficients were as follows:

| Melodic Line | .85 |
|---|---|
| Phrase Length | .90 |
| Articulatory Agility | .90 |
| Grammatical Form | .90 |
| Paraphasia in Running Speech | .79 |
| Word-Finding | .78 |

The High-Probability Repetition subtest was found to have a reliability coefficient of .90, and the four subtests comprising the auditory comprehension scale subtests have reliability coefficients of .96, .68, .91 and .89, thus ensuring an adequate reliability for this scale.

The relatively low reliability of the Word-Finding and Paraphasia ratings corresponds to the subjective uncertainty of the judges in making these ratings. In view of the method of obtaining the reliability coefficients, however, it is felt that they are minimal estimates and that we are on safe ground in having the individual examiner make each rating.

## ADMINISTRATION OF SUBTESTS

With a few exceptions, the subtests of this aphasia examination are scaled so that each begins with easy items and progresses to more difficult ones. The examiner should discontinue testing in each subtest at the point at which it is apparent that no further score can be obtained and that the patient is being stressed by successive failures. There is no objection to aiding the patient by providing the first sound of a response when he is clearly unable to respond without help. Of course, score credit is allowed only for unassisted responses. On the other hand, there is no objection to continuing subtests in the face of successive failure if the patient is unaware of his errors and not bothered by them.

It is also permissible to vary the order of the subtests, if it appears that the patient's motivation will be improved by interspersing subtests that he can do well among those that tap a difficult and frustrating function.

## AUDITORY COMPREHENSION

### Word Discrimination

This is a multiple-choice, auditory word-recognition test. It samples six semantic categories of words: objects, geometric forms, letters, actions, numbers, and colors, giving the opportunity to observe selective impairment of word categories. This test correlates best with the other three auditory comprehension scores (.83 with Body-Part Identification, .80 with Commands, and .69 with Complex Ideational Material).

ADMINISTRATION AND SCORING. Each of the two test cards presents three categories of visual stimuli, and the examiner names items in random rotation among these three categories, forcing the subject to shift his category-set with each test word. Card 2 (Objects, Letters, Forms) is presented first, then Card 3 (Actions, Colors, Numbers). The stimulus question is always in the form, "Show me (slight pause) _____." Scoring allows full credit of two points for correct identification within 5 seconds, partial credit of one point for correct identification after more than 5 seconds (self-correction is permitted), partial credit of half a point for location of the correct category (Column "Cat." on record sheet). If the patient does not locate the correct category, he is directed to it on the card and, if he then succeeds, is allowed partial credit of

half a point (under Column "Cue"). One half point for "Cat." is allowed whether the subject points to the wrong member of the correct category or merely points in the correct group without making a choice. The examiner should record all incorrect choices in writing. The maximum score possible is 72. (This subtest is not scaled and should not be discontinued without trying at least two items of each category.)

### Body-Part Identification

Because of the frequent selective disturbance of body-part comprehension, a larger, separate sampling of this group of words is included. The first 18 items sample a wide range of difficulty in body-part names, including 3 fingers (middle, index, and thumb). Eight items are included for right-left comprehension. This subtest's highest three intercorrelations are within the auditory comprehension cluster: .83 with Word Discrimination, .84 with Commands, and .70 with Complex Ideational Material.

ADMINISTRATION AND SCORING. The patient is asked to point on his own body to the part named by the examiner, with the command, "Show me your (slight pause) _____." While finger identification and right-left discrimination are not scored separately, they deserve special attention as a screening test for disorders of parietal lobe function, in which these concepts may be selectively disturbed. (A more exhaustive test of Finger Identification and Right-Left Discrimination appears in Chapter 6 as part of an assessment of spatial and computational functions.)

Full credit of one point is allowed for each of the first 18 items, if identified within 5 seconds; one-half point is allowed for response of over 5 seconds' latency. Up to 2 additional points are earned for right-left comprehension, for a total possible raw score of 20. In scoring Right-Left Discrimination, only the side of the body is relevant. The patient may point to his right eye instead of "right cheek" without loss of credit.

### Commands

In this subtest, the capacity to process increasingly concentrated auditory information is tested with commands ranging from one significant informational unit to five. Carrying out commands and even pointing, as required in the preceding subtest, presuppose the preservation of the ability to carry out purposeful movements, i.e., the absence of severe *apraxia*. Since apraxia often accompanies aphasia, this possible source of contamination must be borne in mind, particularly if the patient does disproportionately well in the next subtest, which requires only the answering of "yes-no" questions. The highest intercorrelations of this subtest are also within the auditory comprehension cluster: .80 with Word Discrimination, .69 with Complex Ideational Material, and .84 with Body-Part Identification.

ADMINISTRATION AND SCORING. Each command may be repeated once, on request; however, the command must be repeated as a whole. Each underlined element in each command in the test booklet may be passed or failed independently, permitting a score of 0 to 15. (This subtest may be discontinued after two totally failed items.)

### Complex Ideational Material

This subtest requires the patient to understand and express agreement or disagreement concerning factual material that does not relate to a stimulus immediately before him. Starting with simple facts ("Will a cork sink in water?" "Will a stone sink in water?"), the material increases in length and in the demand for reference to knowledge or easy inferences beyond the mere recall of the words. Thus there is an intellectual component, which, however, does not go beyond average adult ability, even at the most difficult level. The intercorrelations with other subtests are highest (.69-.70) with the other three auditory comprehension subtests.

ADMINISTRATION AND SCORING. Each item consists of a pair of questions, one requiring "yes" and the other "no." We have changed the order of the questions from that of the 1972 edition, in order to avoid having subjects automatically give the opposite answer to the second part of a question pair after having said "yes" or "no" to the first part.

In the new sequence, questions 1a through

4a are presented in order, followed by questions 1b through 4b. Both parts "a" and "b" of each numbered item must be answered correctly to earn credit for the item.

Items 5 through 12 are based on the comprehension of four paragraphs, read aloud to the patient. Each paragraph is immediately followed by two pairs of questions. In the new sequence, questions 5a and 6a are followed by 5b and 6b. As before, both halves of each numbered item must be answered correctly. The same procedure applies to items 7 and 8, 9 and 10, and 11 and 12, each set following its respective paragraph.

One point is allowed for each item, with both questions correctly answered, for a maximum of 12 points. (This subtest may be discontinued after four totally failed items.)

## ORAL EXPRESSION

This section begins with the testing of the mechanics of articulation and proceeds from a test of automatized "nonpropositional" speech, through repetition, to progressively more information-carrying acts of word-finding. While tests of sentence repetition and sentence reading are included, the formulation of connected speech is not tested here, but must be evaluated from the conversational and expository speech samples. The final subtest is a measure of word-production fluency in controlled association.

### Nonverbal Agility

This subtest is aimed at providing a comparison between nonverbal use of the lips and tongue as opposed to articulation in actual speech. Contrary to widely held opinion, this correlation is not great. The test consists of a set of six alternating movements, such as protruding and retracting the tongue repeatedly, or alternately pursing and releasing the lips. Poor performance here reflects incoordination and weakness of the speech musculature, which contributes to the nonaphasic dysarthria, which may complicate the symptom complex in some patients. Correlations with the remainder of the language subtests are low, except for a correlation of .62 with Mechanics of Writing.

ADMINISTRATION AND SCORING. Each movement is done after a verbal instruction and demonstration. Full credit of 2 points or half credit of 1 point depends on the number of full alternations done in 5 seconds, timed by the second hand of a watch. The maximum score is 12.

### Verbal Agility

Because of the facilitation afforded by repetition, single-word repetition tests are often well done by patients whose natural speech is dysarthric. On the other hand, these tests may be failed by "fluent" aphasics, who produce paraphasic distortions on repetition.

The approach of this subtest is to bypass both of these sources of error. First, by timing the rate of serial repetitions of the same word, defects that are inaudible in a single-word repetition are reflected in the slowing of serial performance. Second, by aiding the patient to attain initial correct repetition, we overcome the spuriously low scores in articulation that are due to paraphasia. This subtest correlates with rating scale measures of fluency, Automatized Sequences, and the repetition subtests.

ADMINISTRATION AND SCORING. Some patients may be aided in getting started by seeing the written word. Card 4 is provided for this purpose, and the examiner points to each word as it is presented orally. When a patient is prevented by paraphasia or poor comprehension from correctly initiating his repetitions, the item is invalidated. Rejection of more than two items for this reason invalidates the score of this subtest, which may then be discontinued.

Two points or one point per item are earned, depending on the number of correct repetitions of the test word within a 5-second interval. The maximum score is 14. If one or two items are invalidated, prorate the score on the basis of 7/5 or 7/6, as appropriate.

SCORING OF ARTICULATION AND PARAPHASIA. Seven of the following subtests provide for a tally of articulatory difficulty and paraphasic errors for each response. Paraphasia and articulatory difficulty (dysarthria) are mutually exclusive classifications. While there are "gray areas" in which a decision between them is difficult, the principle underlying the two concepts is important to master.

Articulatory difficulty refers to loss of accuracy in forming individual phonemes, so that the sounds that emerge—particularly difficult consonants and blends—are not standard English phonemes. This usually occurs in a context of effort, awkwardness, and slowness of speech. Occasionally, one hears, "infantilisms," such as "ts" for "ch" or "w" for "r." It is in relation to "literal paraphasia" that the confusion with dysarthria is most likely. In the case of literal paraphasia, individual phonemes and syllables are easily produced and are perceived by the listener as standard English phonemes, but their selection and ordering in a word is incorrect.

In scoring, responses that are correct in content receive a tally under the appropriate articulation column:

Normal

Stiff but correct: no transcribable phonemic error, but perceptibly awkward.

Distorted: at least one definite phonemic distortion, but word still recognizable.

Failure: not recognizable due to articulatory difficulty, but considered as an attempt at the target word.

Paraphasic errors should be tallied even when self corrected. The four columns on the right side of the page provide an opportunity to tally paraphasia under four headings. The first three columns on the right refer to paraphasic errors referable to known target words.

1. *Neologistic Distortion*—Introduction of extraneous phonemes or transposition of intended phonemes so that less than half of the intended word is discernible as an intact unit. In the extreme, distortions may take the form of neologistic nonwords.
2. *Literal Paraphasia*—Transposition or introduction of extraneous phonemes such that more than half of the intended word is produced as an intact unit.
3. *Verbal Paraphasia*—Substitution of an inappropriate word during the effort to say a particular target word. Perseveration of a previously used word is in-

cluded here, but only once for any per-severated word.

4. *Other*—A number of types of paraphasia that involve extended speech sequences. It also is used for some types of non-paraphasic, inappropriate responses, defined in the following. The abbreviation of the category should be written into the column.

npg—neologistic paragrammatism: running speech including neologistic expressions, usually with some real English words (referred to as "extended neologistic jargon" in the first edition)

pg—paragrammatism: running speech composed of English words in a semantically or grammatically unacceptable sequence (referred to as "extended English jargon" in the first edition)

irrel.—irrelevant speech that is not paraphasic, but inappropriate

cl.—circumlocution

The use of recurrent stereotyped syllables or words is not scored as paraphasia.

The total number of paraphasias checked under each column is totalled for the oral-expression subtests from Automatized Sequences through Body-Part Naming and entered on the Subtest Summary Profile. The pattern of the breakdown of paraphasias, particularly the relative incidence of literal paraphasia, contributes to the diagnostic classification. (See Chapter 7 for a discussion of syndromes and case illustrations.)

### Automatized Sequences

In this subtest, four well-overlearned sequences are tested: days of the week, months of the year, numbers from 1 to 21 and the alphabet. Recitation of memorized sequences is commonly better preserved than propositional speech, and this is usually true for aphasics of all types. Especially dramatic discrepancies in favor of recitation are found in transcortical aphasics (see Chapter 7). Correlations ranging from .60 to .76 are observed with verbal agility and the repetition tests.

ADMINISTRATION AND SCORING. Many patients succeed only when the first word is supplied, and no credit is lost for help in initiating

a series. The patient may be assisted by prompting in the middle of a series, but no more than four items should be supplied before discontinuing. The test booklet shows from three to nine words per line, and this *may* lead to multiple entries of articulation and paraphasia on each line. No more than one check should be entered in any column, but as many different columns as are needed may be checked to record the level of articulation and types of paraphasia produced with the words on a given line.

Two points maximum are allowed for complete recitation of any series, whether or not the initial word was supplied by the examiner. One point partial credit is allowed for unaided runs of consecutive words of various lengths as follows: days—four consecutive; months—five consecutive; numbers—eight consecutive; alphabet—seven consecutive; maximum score is 8.

### Recitation, Singing, and Rhythm

The trio of performances sampled in this section were grouped together because of their apparent relationship to musical ability; however, intercorrelations between them are low. Reciting "nursery rhymes" has correlation coefficients in the .50s, with scores based on word and sentence repetition, but rhythm-tapping and melody are largely independent of language skills and are only slightly related to each other. While, clinically, the ability to sing a melody correctly is usually preserved in severe aphasics, the ability to produce the words with the melody is much less common and characterizes "transcortical" aphasics, in whom the remarkable preservation of verbal recitation is associated with selective sparing of repetition.

Thus, while the presumed common contribution of these three performances to musical ability is unproved, we have continued to group them in a single section, with three separate rating-scale scores.

ADMINISTRATION AND SCORING. *Recitation.* Several nursery rhymes are suggested to elicit completion responses. Occasionally, a patient takes offense at being presented with childish content, but this reaction can be avoided by explaining, "Many of our patients who have trouble talking find it easy to say things they learned when they were very young. I am going to let you hear some nursery rhymes that you probably remember, and see if you can go on where I leave off." It is suggested that the Lord's Prayer be tried as an alternative, or in addition, to the nursery rhymes.

Score 0—If the patient can complete no line of verse.

Score 1—If the patient can complete at least one line of verse on any of the trials.

Score 2—If the patient can complete at least two verses unaided or three with a cue.

*Melody.* Since many adults are reticent about singing alone, the examiner should start the song, encouraging the patient by gesture to join, and then sing softly enough to hear how accurately the patient carries the melody. If the patient has a preferred song, he may sing that instead of "My country 'tis of thee" (America).

Score 0—If the patient is amelodic or sings melody totally unrelated to the target.

Score 1—If the melody is recognizable, although it may be inaccurate and incompletely recalled.

Score 2—If the melody is essentially accurate.

*Tapping Rhythms.* Four rhythmic patterns are tapped with a pencil by the examiner for the patient to imitate. The first three are simple cyclic patterns, which are tapped over and over through six cycles: first: ⌣′ ⌣′ ⌣′ second: ′⌣⌣ ′⌣⌣ third: ⌣′′ ⌣′′. The fourth is the familiar rhythm of the jingle, "Shave and a haircut, two bits": ′⌣⌣′′,′′.

Score 0—If the patient reproduces no rhythms.

Score 1—If the patient reproduces at least one of the rhythms.

Score 2—If the patient imitates all rhythms.

### Repetition of Words

Word repetition is an easy task, and only the most severely impaired patients fail it completely. Failure may be due to poor comprehension, as is frequently the case in Wernicke's aphasia and even more so in the rare instances of word-deafness. The arousal of a fragment of the auditory image will be reflected in well-articulated, but paraphasic, responses in which a fragment of the word can be identified. Occasionally, the sound of the stimulus word appears to be lost immediately, while the patient has grasped and retained some of its meaning. His effort to repeat emerges as a verbal paraphasia, i.e., a word related by connotation to the stimulus.

Another source of failure to repeat is severe incapacitation of the motor speech output system, auditory word recognition being adequate. In such cases, speech output is reduced to little more than a few highly overlearned expressions, if that. Of course, loss of comprehension may coexist with impaired motor output, so that careful exploration is needed before ascribing a cause to failure of repetition.

Finally, repetition failure may occur with fluent spontaneous speech and normal auditory comprehension in *conduction aphasia.* In this disorder, literal paraphasia interferes with repetition, but rarely at the level of single common English words. The highest correlations of this subtest are with Automatized Sequences (.76), with High-Probability Repetition (.73), and with Verbal Agility (.75).

ADMINISTRATION AND SCORING. In this subtest, a wide sampling of word types is presented, including a grammatical function word, objects, colors, a letter, numbers, an abstract verb of three syllables, and a tongue twister ("Methodist Episcopal"). The order of the first five words has been changed, but the stimuli are the same as in the first edition (1972 version). Notation of articulation and paraphasia is made in the appropriate column. An item is scored correct if all phonemes are in correct order and recognizable. One point is allowed per item for a total of ten points.

### Repeating Phrases and Sentences

This section is divided into two separately scored sets of sentences, differing in vocabulary difficulty and predictability of the verbal content, and referred to as "high-probability" and "low-probability" sentences. For example, at the five-word level, a high-probability sentence is, "You should not tell her"; a low-probability sentence is, "Pry the tin lid off." The separation of the test into two sets is based on previous findings that showed that patients with severe anomic aphasia have an enormous overdependence on the predictability of the content, with resulting discrepancies between high- and low-probability scores. Nevertheless, the correlation between the two scores is fairly high (.86). Since repetition of sentences is a complex operation depending on many components, the diagnostic significance of this subtest depends on its relation to other performances. When it is deviantly high in comparison with naming and comprehension, it indicates transcortical aphasia; when deviantly low in comparison with phrase length and comprehension, it indicates conduction aphasia.

ADMINISTRATION AND SCORING. The sentences must be read as an uninterrupted unit for patient to repeat, alternating between a high-probability and a low-probability item. For credit on any item, all words must be reproduced without paraphasic errors, but articulatory distortions consistent with the patient's general articulatory difficulty are not penalized.

One point is allowed for each sentence correctly repeated and high- and low-probability sections are scored separately from zero to eight.

## Word Reading

This is a test of word finding that is, however, dependent on basic reading ability. If subsequent testing shows that the patient no longer recognizes written language, this score must be interpreted purely in that light. It is possible, however, for the written word to be understood and failed orally for two reasons. The meaning may be grasped or partially grasped without arousing a phonologic component sufficient to guide the final speech output. In this case, the patient may respond with a word related in meaning to the stimulus, e.g., saying "green" for "brown" or "square" for "circle." Alternatively, he may associate phonetically to part of a word, with

or without grasping its meaning, e.g., saying "char" for "chair." On the other hand, he may fully appreciate the phonetic structure of the stimulus, yet fail because of inability to mobilize the motor speech system, as in the case of the patient who can articulate few words under any conditions.

As a test of word finding, word reading is easier than confrontation naming for some patients because the written word directly arouses phonetic associations without the necessity for mediation by comprehension, or the intent to express the meaning of the word. Understandably, the .87 correlation with Visual Confrontation Naming is on a par with that for Oral Sentence Reading (.78).

ADMINISTRATION AND SCORING. The words are read from Card 5 as the examiner exposes them one at a time, by using a card as a place marker to shield the rest of the list. Full credit is allowed for response within 3 seconds and partial credit for response in 3 to 10 seconds or 10 to 30 seconds. The examiner checks under the column heading corresponding to the time delay. The examiner's estimate of the delay gives sufficient precision in scoring. (The use of a stopwatch is unnecessarily cumbersome.) Paraphasia and articulation are to be checked for each response. The maximum score of 30 is based on 3 points full credit on each item. Partial credits are summed according to the response delay indicated in the column heading in which response is recorded. Discontinue only if the first four words are failed.

## Responsive Naming

In this approach to word finding, an orally presented question serves as the stimulus. The response words include nouns (watch, scissors, match, drugstore), colors (green, black), verbs (shave, wash, write) and a number (twelve). While performance here obviously depends on a certain minimum of auditory comprehension, its closest correlation is with Visual Confrontation Naming (.87). This supports the concept of word finding as a separate component of language, whether stimulus input is by spoken word or picture. When the percentile score for performance on this test is much below that for Visual Confrontation Naming, it is usually due to impaired auditory comprehension.

It should be noted that the stimulus questions usually contain a key word that is a close associate of the expected response. For those patients who have exceptionally strong verbal-associative skills, performance in this task may exceed that for Visual Confrontation Naming.

ADMINISTRATION AND SCORING. As in the other naming subtests, the score depends on the time interval required to produce the response. A check is entered for any correct response, under the column heading (0–3″, 3–10″, 10–30″) corresponding to the approximate response delay, as estimated by the examiner. In case of a paraphasic response, the record should show what was said and a tally check entered in the appropriate paraphasia column. For correct responses, the quality of articulation should be entered. Total the number of points (3, 2, 1, or 0) corresponding to the columns that are checked. The maximum score possible is 30.

### Visual Confrontation Naming

Naming to visual presentation is a universally used test for aphasia since virtually all aphasic patients have some loss of capacity to perform. While it may be described as a visual input/oral output task, there is reason to believe that this is a simplistic view that does not do justice to the intervening processes. The form taken by the errors gives some inkling as to where and how the naming process is going astray. Thus, patients whose difficulty is primarily at the speech-output stage are likely to show difficulties in articulation that are relieved by having the word supplied by the examiner. They are self critical and discriminate sharply between the correct and erroneous response. Those who fail to evoke the correct premotor phonologic pattern are more likely to produce paraphasic mistakes. When the correct word is offered them, it may not register as correct, even though their auditory comprehension is excellent in other contexts. Thus, there is evidence in some patients of a two-way dissociation between the concept and the word. Patients whose paraphasia is confined to phonemic substitutions

and transpositions are usually acutely aware of their errors, but have the same difficulty when offered the word for repetition. These are the "conduction aphasics," discussed in Chapter 7.

The stimulus items on Cards 2 and 3 are the same ones used in the word-discrimination test, and include objects, geometric forms, letters, actions, numbers, colors, and body parts. Three additional body parts have been added to this subtest. The examiner points to the body part to be named.

The various categories are often unevenly affected by aphasia. Letter naming and number naming are most often spared, while object naming is least often spared (Goodglass, Klein, Carey, and Jones, 1966). While, for quantitative purposes, the total score is the only measure of achievement on this test, the examiner should attend to the previously mentioned qualitative features, i.e., relationship among the word categories, category of paraphasia, if any, and response to assistance in saying intended words.

ADMINISTRATION AND SCORING. The examiner estimates the reaction time for each correct response and enters a check in the column labeled with the corresponding time interval. The maximum score obtainable for the 38 items is 114. Paraphasias should be tallied and entered verbatim for later reference. Articulation level should be tallied for all correct responses. (Since this subtest is not scaled, do not discontinue without trying at least one item from each category.)

### Animal Naming (Fluency in Controlled Association)

A further approach to word finding is that of measuring fluency in controlled association. This is a widely used technique in clinical testing, and it appears in two forms in the Stanford-Binet: once in the form of unrestricted word naming and once in the form of animal naming. The procedure suggested here is an adaptation of the Stanford-Binet procedure for animal naming, modified by giving the subject preliminary instructions to consider animals of all varieties and finally giving a starting word, "dog." The purpose of these instructions is to facilitate the task in two ways: first, to provide a preliminary set that may assist the subject in shifting from one category to another, and, second, to provide a definite starting point for timing, since many aphasics have inordinate difficulty in initiating a chain of associations, yet have reasonable fluency once under way.

The norm for 10-year-old children is 12 different animals in 60 seconds. Average adults name about 18. Performance in this type of test is reduced not only in aphasics, but in many brain-injured patients whose speed of mental processes and ability to shift are impaired. While most normal subjects start off naming rapidly in the first 15 seconds, then taper off, aphasics more frequently run out of associations early and recover repeatedly with another burst of words.

This subtest has its highest correlation (.70) with Visual Confrontation Naming, and a correlation of .69 with Responsive Naming.

ADMINISTRATION AND SCORING. The instructions to the patient are given in the wording provided in the test booklet, and the examiner starts timing when he provides "dog" as the first word. Words are listed under the 15-second grouping columns provided in the test booklet, and 90 seconds are allowed for naming. The score consists of the number of different words named in the most productive consecutive 60-second period, not counting the examiner's starting word.

### Oral Sentence Reading

Reading connected material aloud goes beyond the requirements for reading detached words in that it places a demand on the patient's command of grammatical forms. The small grammatical words and inflectional endings are often omitted by those patients who omit them in spontaneous speech. This complex task is included, not so much because of its value as an analytic technique, but because the interaction of many component factors makes this peformance difficult to predict unless it is tested directly. For example, a high degree of accomplishment in phonetic association may overcome a severe aphasia and result in surprisingly good performance. The word-reading test is subject to the same

underlying skill and, naturally enough, these tests correlate strongly (.78).

ADMINISTRATION AND SCORING. Sentences are read from Cards 6 and 7. A sentence-reading task offers great temptation to allow partial credit for nearly correct performance. Because this would raise as many scoring problems as it would solve, a simple all-or-none score was decided on for each sentence. No credit is lost for articulatory awkwardness that is consistent with the patient's speech, but no transpositions of sounds or other paraphasic intrusions are permitted. Score zero to ten, one point per sentence. (Discontinue after three failures.)

## UNDERSTANDING WRITTEN LANGUAGE

The subtests of this section focus on a number of the elementary associative skills that either underlie reading or are byproducts of the way we learn to read. For example, recognition of the equivalence of letters written in various styles is a necessary and universal accomplishment of the normal reader, while recognition of oral spelling is a byproduct, not a part, of the normal reading process, yet one that is a sign of the intactness of the reading apparatus. Comprehension of connected material is tested by an untimed multiple-choice test. There is no attempt to measure speed and efficiency at the upper levels of reading skill, where a speed test would encroach on the range of normal adult reading ability.

### Symbol and Word Discrimination

A prerequisite to reading comprehension is the recognition of letters as familiar symbols, apart from recalling their names or phonetic value. Our means of testing this function is the multiple-choice matching of letters and short words across different styles of writing—upper- and lower-case, cursive and printed. This is a purely visual recognition task, yet its intimate relationship with the mechanics of reading is demonstrated by the fact that its highest correlation (.67) is with the task of matching pictures to written words. The next four highest correlations are within the group of reading subtests. In difficulty, it is on a low level, and missing more than one item usually corresponds to severe reading difficulty.

ADMINISTRATION AND SCORING. The two Cards, 8 and 9, contain the ten items. In each case, the examiner points to the model word or letter centered above the five multiple-choice responses and asks the subject to select the equivalent. If the patient's auditory comprehension is defective, he may usually be led to understand by pantomime, using the first item as a demonstration. Scoring is one point per item, for a maximum of ten. This subtest is not scaled and should be given in its entirety, unless the patient cannot grasp the instructions.

## Phonetic Association

The link between sound and letter is tested by two procedures separately scored, Word Recognition and Comprehension of Oral Spelling.

WORD RECOGNITION. This subtest was designed to reveal the intactness of auditory-visual phonetic associations without necessarily involving either comprehension or verbalization by the patient. The task is to select, from a multiple choice of five written words, the one spoken by the examiner. A second feature is built into this task that occasionally reveals a striking phenomenon—the ability to respond to the connotative meaning of a written word *without* appreciating its phonetic value. Examination of the multiple-choice sets shows that in four items the incorrect choices consist of three words connotatively similar to the test word and only one word similar in structure. Thus, for the second item, "pond," the four incorrect words are "lake," "water," "creek," and "fond." In the remaining four items, the proportion is reversed, i.e., three words are structurally similar and one is related by meaning. For example, for the first item, "ship," the four incorrect choices are "shop," "slip," "skip," and "boat." While the ability to associate between a concept and a written word without an inner phonetic experience is occasionally found at the one-word level, there is evidence that normal reading does involve phonologic mediation. The intercorrelations of this subtest are primarily within the reading cluster, with the highest

correlation of .66 with Word-Picture Matching.

*Administration and Scoring.* Using Cards 10 and 11, the examiner instructs the patient to find the one word, out of five on a line, that matches the word the examiner says. The words are given in the order in which they appear in the test booklet. Score one point for each correct answer for a maximum of eight.

COMPREHENSION OF ORAL SPELLING. Understanding orally spelled words is obviously not a part of the normal reading process. We might question its relevance in aphasia entirely, were it not true that (1) it is universally acquired in the usual course of acquisition of written language and (2) it is a fragile skill in the face of some cases of aphasia, even with patients who read adequately on written presentation. While this task demands the participation of auditory comprehension, it has correlations in the .60s, not only within the auditory comprehension cluster, but with tests of naming, repetition, and writing.

*Administration and Scoring.* The patient is asked to listen while a word is spelled aloud to him and then immediately to say or otherwise indicate what it is. The words should be spelled at about two letters per second. If the patient appears to recognize a word but cannot express it, it may be offered as a multiple choice, with several similar-sounding words, for him to identify. The multiple-choice procedure is open to guesswork, for it may permit the patient to identify a spelled word that he only partially recognized. While a score obtained by multiple choice has some uncertainty, the examiner may judge the range of uncertainty. One point is allowed for each correct recognition for a maximum score of eight points. (Discontinue if the first three items are failed.)

## Word-Picture Matching

This is the first subtest in which comprehension of the meaning of written words is involved. The ten words selected (on Card 5) correspond to objects, actions, colors, numbers, and geometric forms appearing on Cards 2 and 3. These are the same words that were used earlier in the testing of auditory word discrimination, naming, and oral word reading. This task may be performed well by patients whose poor auditory comprehension has caused them to fail on the preceding pair of subtests. Understanding individual words is a prerequisite for comprehension of any written sentences. The highest intercorrelations of this subtest are within the cluster of reading tasks: .66 with Word Recognition, .73 with Reading Sentences and Paragraphs, and .67 with Symbol and Word Discrimination.

ADMINISTRATION AND SCORING. The test words are printed on Card 5, while the corresponding pictures to be identified are on Cards 2 and 3. Card 5 is slipped under the appropriate picture card in such a way that the edge of the picture-stimulus card acts as a line guide for each successive test word, and the subject is instructed to point to the picture (or number or color or form) corresponding to the word. Card 5 is slipped from Card 2 to Card 3 as called for by the location of the test picture. The score is based on one point per correct match for a maximum of ten.

### Reading Sentences and Paragraphs

Some patients show an abrupt failure at the simplest levels of sentence comprehension, although they read well at the one-word level. As in the case of oral sentence reading, we are dealing here with a complex task that is most difficult to predict from performances in other more elementary tasks. Hence, this subtest primarily serves the purpose of describing the level of functioning in an important linguistic skill, rather than pointing to an elementary component of language that may help explain more complex functions. While the highest correlation is with Word-Picture Matching (.73), there are correlations in the .60s with tests of Auditory Comprehension and of Writing.

The technique of sentence completion with a four-way multiple choice is easy to convey to the patient and much less subject to guesswork than the true-false question. The choice of possible answers always includes several wrong responses that are associatively related to words in the stimulus material. Thus, it is not possible to pass these questions merely by noting a salient word and selecting an asso-

ciate to it. The range is from first-grade to high-school level difficulty in a ten-item scale.

ADMINISTRATION AND SCORING. Use Cards 12 through 16. Two buffer items are provided, and the examiner may read one or both of these aloud, as he considers necessary, pointing to each of the choices in turn, for the patient to indicate his selection. The examiner underlines the patient's choice in the test booklet. The first regular item is then administered without any help in the form of oral reading, although the examiner may, for impaired patients, point to the words in the test sentence and to the sequence of choices. One point is allowed for each correct answer for a maximum of ten points. (Discontinue after three failures.)

## WRITING

The examination of writing is analogous to that of speech, in that we examine the mechanics of writing movements, the recall of written symbols for execution through various modes of stimulation, and the formulation of connected material in free narrative and from dictation. These correspond to the levels of articulation, word finding, and formulation of connected discourse in speech.

### Mechanics of Writing

The scoring of Mechanics of Writing has been redefined. It is now to be based on a review of all of the patients' written output, including signature and address, transcription of the "Quick brown fox" sentence, Spelling to Dictation, Written Confrontation Naming, Sentences to Dictation, and Narrative Writing. The reason for this change is that patients who could copy the "Quick brown fox" sentence only in a slavish manner in block letters were frequently found to use fairly good cursive writing in dictation or other noncopying tasks. In order to obtain norms with the revised scale, 100 protocols were rescored on the basis of the new standards. The intercorrelations, however, are based on the original scoring. As in the 1972 computations, correlations between Mechanics of Writing and other language tasks are low, even within the writing cluster, in which the highest correlation is .52, with Serial Writing. Although the rating is applied after all the writing tasks have been attempted, the first procedure in the Writing section is still to obtain a signature and transcription of a model sentence, since some patients can perform only at this level.

ADMINISTRATION AND SCORING. The patient is instructed to write his name and address using his more able hand. If he fails, these are block printed by the examiner, and the patient is instructed to transcribe them into his own writing or, failing that, to copy them. The patient is then required to copy the printed sentence in the test booklet into his own handwriting or, if that is not possible, to copy in the same form. Scoring is deferred until the patient has done all the remaining writing subtests of which he is capable. Performance is scored only with respect to the recall of the movements of letter formation on the basis of the following five-point scale:

1. No legible letters.
2. Occasional success on single letters (block printing).
3. Block printing with some malformed letters.
4. Legible but impaired cursive writing and/or upper- and lower-case printing.
5. Judged to be the same as premorbid writing, with allowance made for use of nonpreferred hand.

### Recall of Written Symbols

This subtest is divided into two separately scored sections: (1) *Serial Writing*—alphabet and numbers to 21 and (2) *Primer-Level Dictation*—writing individual numbers, letters, and primer words to dictation. This represents the easiest level of written symbol recall—a level that does not yet involve any communication of meaning. The association of the written response to the dictated stimulus does not necessarily imply the intermediation of comprehension. The two sections have an intercorrelation of .80.

ADMINISTRATION AND SCORING. In part one, Serial Writing, the patient is instructed to write the alphabet and then to write numbers up to twenty-one. If he does not understand, the first 3 items of each set may be

written to start him off. The score is the total number of different, correct letters and numbers, combined for a maximum score of 47. In part two, *Primer-Level Dictation*, the letters, numbers, and primer words in the test booklet are dictated, and the score is the combined total correct (up to 15) on these 3 sets.

### Written Word Finding

This subtest taps the written vocabulary beyond the primer level, in the range of words of average difficulty. It, too, is divided into two subsections: (1) *Spelling to Dictation* and (2) *Written Confrontation Naming*.

SPELLING TO DICTATION. Performance requires writing a list of ten dictated words. Spelling from dictation is theoretically possible without the intervention of the comprehension of meaning. Some individuals show a strongly automatized phonetic association between auditory input and spelled output. It is of interest to ask patients to spell orally words that they fail to write. Provision is made in the test booklet to record this information, but it is not scored.

Oral spelling appears to be partly autonomous from the written performance. Many individuals have the knack of rattling off oral spelling rapidly without much success in using this to guide their written spelling. Oral spelling calls on auditory-verbal imagery and purely temporal sequencing, aided by highly overlearned sequential probabilities among the letters of English words. This contrasts with the requirement of spatial sequencing in writing, and with the fact that the slowness of writing greatly reduces the benefits of overlearned temporal sequences in the motor-kinesthetic sphere.

The correlation of spelling with other subtests is highest (.85) with Written Confrontation Naming and (.77) with Sentences to Dictation.

*Administration and Scoring.* The words are presented orally, with clear enunciation, and the patient is required to write them on a clean sheet of paper. The test may be discontinued at the discretion of the examiner if the patient is clearly beyond his depth. If there are any words failed in writing, the patient should be asked to spell them aloud. Score written spelling only. Note additional success in oral spelling for qualitative interpretation.

WRITTEN CONFRONTATION NAMING. This is the first subtest in which the patient is asked to convey information in writing. The vocabulary used consists of some of the objects, colors, forms, actions, and numbers previously used to test auditory comprehension, naming, and reading. This test has its strongest intercorrelations within the writing cluster and secondary correlations in the reading comprehension group and with naming.

*Administration and Scoring.* The examiner, using Cards 2 and 3, points *silently* to the items in the order in which they appear in the test booklet. The patient is given paper and pencil and instructed orally or in pantomime to write the names. Score one for each correctly spelled response, for a maximum of ten.

## Written Formulation

In this subtest, we assess the patient's level of function in the complex task of writing connected sentences, first in free narrative about the "cookie theft" scene, then in response to dictation.

NARRATIVE WRITING. This performance is the complex resultant of the ability to find the needed words, to formulate sentences, and to spell. Many patients who can write individual words well are overwhelmed by the task of forming sentences and give up after a feeble effort. Occasionally, one obtains fluent but grossly irrelevant writing, usually from patients who also produce fluent, paraphasic speech. This test correlates well with Sentences to Dictation (.80), with Spelling to Dictation (.75), and with Written Naming (.77). A secondary group of correlations in the .60s is with the naming subtests.

*Administration and Scoring.* The patient is given a fresh sheet of paper, presented with the "cookie theft" picture (Card 1) and instructed to, "Write as much as you can about what you see going on in this picture." He is encouraged to continue writing for 2 minutes, but may be permitted to work longer if his writing is relevant, but exceptionally slow.

The rating scale for scoring narrative writing has been completely redesigned because of the experience that the 1972 scale ratings

did not adequately reflect clinical assessment of performance. The emphasis is on the communication of ideas in writing, given that the mechanics of writing and correctness of spelling are scored elsewhere. There is no penalty for errors of spelling or grammar until the fourth and fifth steps of the scale, which is as follows:

Rating (to be circled)

0—*No relevant words*—Writing is either illegible or paragraphic. There may be some grammatical morphemes, but no recognizable relevant nouns or verbs.

1—*Limited number (1 to 4) of relevant words*—One or more of the nouns or verbs related to the picture are recognizable (even if misspelled). These may appear as isolated words or embedded in a paragraphic string. There are no legible phrases.

2—*One or more phrases*—At least one instance of a word combination forming the nucleus of a phrase, e.g., noun plus verb, subject noun plus object noun. There is no sequence of ideas.

OR

Extensive (five or more) listing of isolated relevant nouns or verbs.

3—*Connected ideas*—At least two actions or descriptive statements in a connected sequence. No penalty for agrammatism or paraphasic errors.

4—*Organized account*—Coherent account with only minor paraphasias, grammatical or spelling errors.

OR

Unduly simplified sentences.

5—*Normal*—Judged normal for patient's estimated premorbid level.

Figure 4 provides illustrations of patient samples to serve as a guide for scoring at each level.

SENTENCES TO DICTATION. While the relatively unstructured writing task of free narrative is beyond the capacity of most aphasics, many of them reveal potential ability when offered preformulated sentences from dictation. The three sentences provided refer to the "cookie theft" picture and are graded in length and grammatical complexity. This sub-

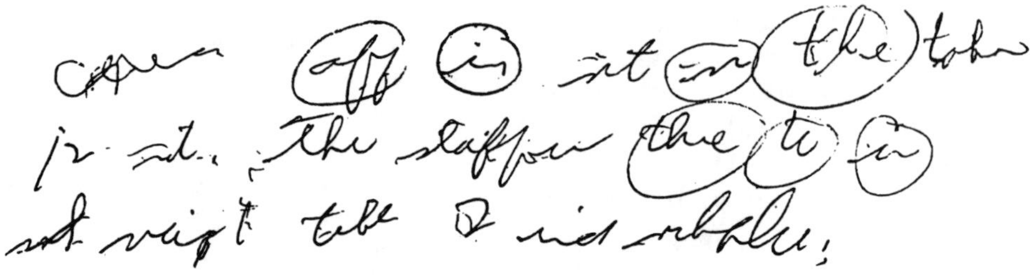

Level 0

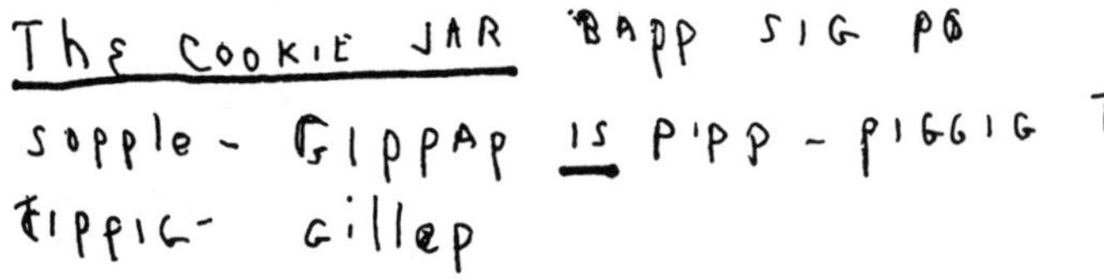

The COOKIE JAR BAPP SIG PB
sopple- GIPPAP IS PIPP - PIGGIG TIGG
TIPPIC- cillep

Level 1

KOOKIE    KOOK    COOK

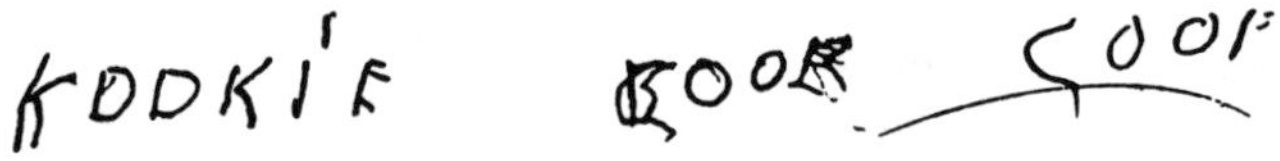

Level 1

DISHES
WATER ON
COOKE.
LIPS

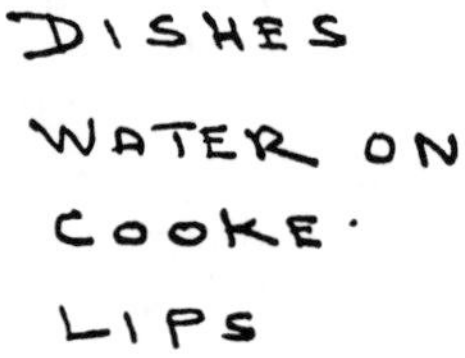

Level 1

**Fig. 4.** Standards for scoring of narrative writing.

*a bay fall off athed ~~sadtl~~ stolla*
*~~the take~~*
*the dished rishoof todg*

Level 2

*girls, boy, woman, ~~food~~ cookie jar*
*stool, dishes, water, faucet*
*cabinet, curtains, cup*
*bowl.*

Level 2

THE BOY IS COMING DOWN WILL
STAIN, BY STEAL WALL THE COOKING.
THE MOTHER IS WASHING THE
~~DINN~~ ("dishes") AND THE WATER IS

("dripping") DOWN.

Level 3

**Fig. 4.** *Continued*

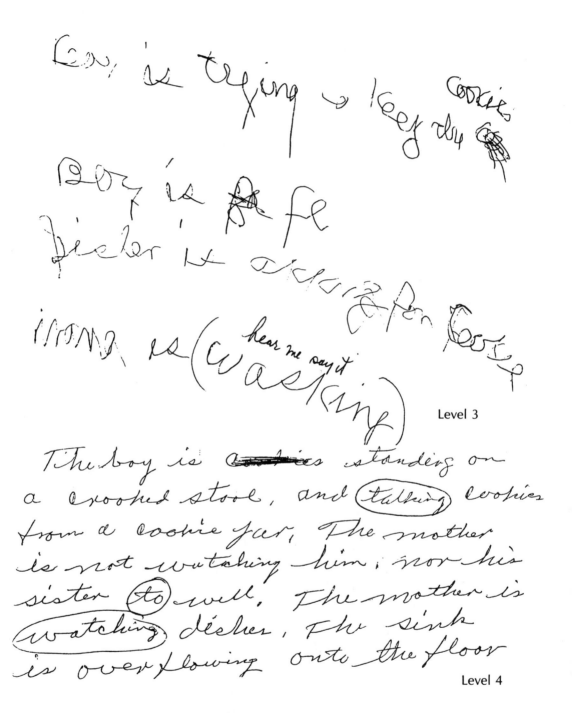

Level 3

Level 4

**Fig. 4.** *Continued*

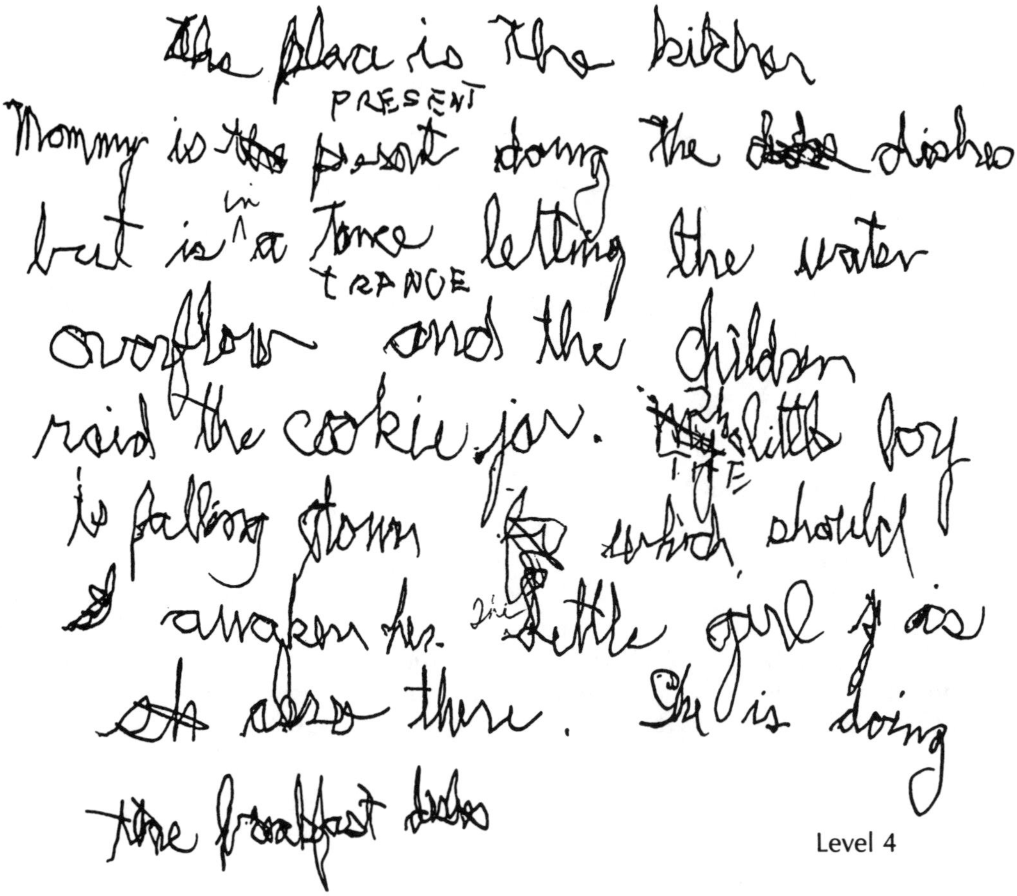

The place is the kitchen
Mommy is the PRESENT present doing the dishes
but is in a Tance TRANCE letting the water
overflow and the children
raid the cookie jar. little boy
is falling down which should
I awaken her. The little girl is
also there. She is doing
the breakfast

Level 4

The boy is standing on the tilting
stool. His mother is washing
the dishes. The water is dripping
all the floor.

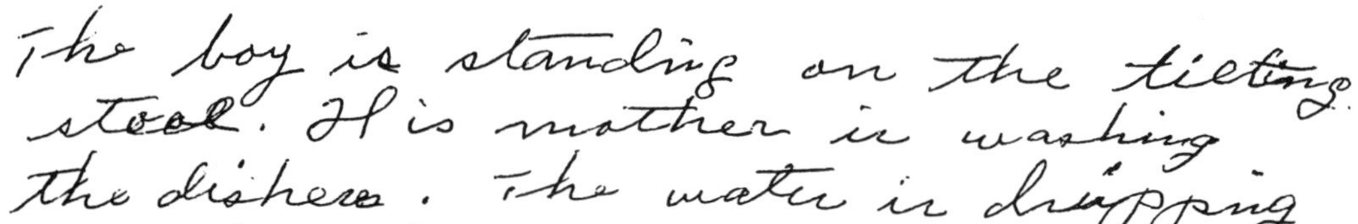

Level 4

**Fig. 4.** *Continued*

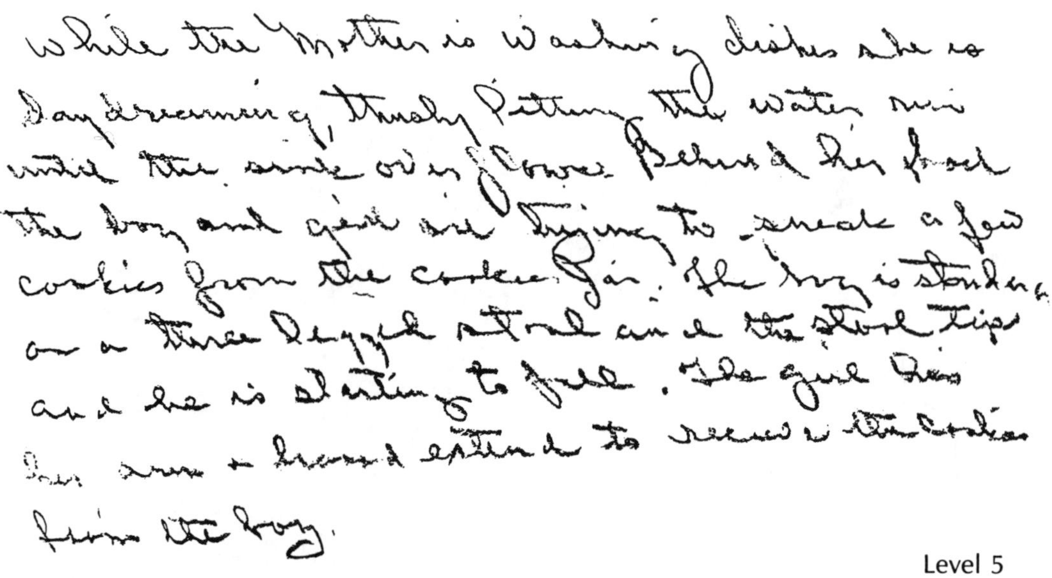

Level 5

**Fig. 4.** *Continued*

test has its highest correlations (.62 to .81) with other writing tasks.

*Administration and Scoring.* The three sentences given in the test booklet are dictated, with no time limit imposed on the patient's writing. Each of the 3 sentences is scored from 0 to 4 points according to the scale in the test booklet, and the subtest score is the total of the 3, for a maximum of 12. Insertion or substitution of irrelevant words is called "paragraphia" and is scored on a 3-point scale as (0) conspicuous, (1) minor, and (2) absent.

# CHAPTER 5

## Supplementary Language Tests

We present here a number of further procedures for the use of the examiner who is interested in a more complete understanding of the patient's language functioning because of its value in diagnosis, therapy, or both. These procedures consist of tests with which there is experimental or clinical experience, but that have not been incorporated into the aphasia battery. They cover an exploration of psycholinguistic factors in auditory comprehension and in expression, exploration of disorders of repetition, study of the sparing of comprehension of whole-body movement commands, and screening for hemispheric disconnection symptoms.

### PSYCHOLINGUISTIC EXPLORATION OF AUDITORY COMPREHENSION

Goodglass, Gleason, and Hyde (1970) presented evidence that impaired auditory comprehension cannot be regarded as an undifferentiated disorder, and that the relative impairment of vocabulary comprehension, span, and prepositional comprehension varies systematically in diagnostic subgroups of patients. Their results agree with Luria's report (1966) that constructions (usually hinging on prepositions) that signal logicogrammatical relationships are impaired in certain forms of aphasia. These, among others, are covered by the items suggested in this section.

#### Prepositions of Location

Invert a cup on the table and give the patient a penny. Sit alongside the patient to elim-

inate ambiguity about "front" and "back" of the cup. Say, "Put the penny *under* the cup. Put the penny *behind* the cup. Put the penny *to the left of* the cup. Put the penny *in front of* the cup. Put the penny *on* the cup. Hold the penny *over* the cup. Put the penny *to the right of* the cup." Place penny a few inches in front of the cup and say, "Move the penny *away* from the cup. Move the penny *toward* the cup." If there is any hesitancy or error, repeat the commands in random order until you can tell which are consistently passed, which are "brittle areas," and which are pure guesswork.

#### "Before"-"After"

Ask for a "yes"-"no" response to the following:

> "Do you eat lunch *after* supper?"
> "Do you eat supper *after* lunch?"
> "Do you put on your shoes *after* your stockings?"
> "Do you put on your stockings *before* your shoes?"
> "Is noontime *before* evening?"
> "Is evening *before* noontime?"

#### "With-To" Pointing

In commands involving manipulation of one object to touch another, the patient may tend to pick up the first object named, regardless of the prepositions "with" and "to" which may tell him to do otherwise.

In the following series, we begin with a

shaping procedure to create the proper performance set, and then use a number of elongated objects (pen, fork, comb), with commands.

*General Instructions:*

Give commands slowly with slight emphasis on the four key words: "with," "to," and the two objects. The item to be picked up is referred to in the following as the "implement," the other as the "object." Partial credit, as explained subsequently, is allowed for lexical errors in the selection of the "object," provided that the "implement" is correctly chosen.

*Materials:* Pen, Fork, Comb

1. Screening

   Verify that the patient can point to any two objects on command in the sequence given (e.g., "Point to the fork, then to the pen."; "Point to the pen, then to the comb."). Assist, if necessary, but the patient must perform twice unaided before proceeding to the Shaping Procedure. If he cannot reach this criterion, terminate test as *"Failed Screening."*

2. Shaping Procedure—Score is based on items "b" through "g."

   a. "Please pick up the comb."

   b. "Now, with the comb, point to the pen."

   If the patient performs adequately, proceed to "c" and count as correct. Otherwise, explain and demonstrate the action. The patient must then perform twice unaided. If he cannot reach this criterion, terminate as "Failed to shape." This item, however, is scored as *incorrect* if assisted.

   c. "Now, point to the pen with the fork."

   If the patient picks up the *pen* to point with, say "Okay, but I said point *to* the pen *with* the fork" while demonstrating the correct action. Count item as incorrect and give no further assistance, but continue through item "g."

3. Unassisted Items: Accept all performances with "Okay" and no other feedback.

   d. "Now, point to the comb with the pen."

   e. "With the comb, point to the fork."

   f. "Point to the pen with the fork."

   g. "Point to the comb with the fork."

*Scoring* (Circle Score):

0—Failed Screening

1—Failed to Shape

2—Fewer than four items correct

3—a. Four of six items totally correct *or* self corrected without assistance.

OR

b. Three items totally correct or self corrected and two more correct with respect to the "implement," but with lexical error on the "object."

4—a. All items correct, but with one or more self corrections.

OR

b. At least four items totally correct or self corrected, with one or two lexical errors on the "object."

5—No errors or self corrections.

## Passive Subject-Object Discrimination

The passive word order (e.g., "The lion was killed by the tiger") reverses the position of agent vs. victim, with respect to the word order expected in the more common active sentence construction. The listener must utilize the particles "was" and "by" to identify agent and victim. Our data indicate this to be a most difficult discrimination for aphasics, who often interpret the sentence on the basis of the active word order, namely, that the agent precedes the verb and the victim follows. In order to examine the comprehension of the passive construction, we present the following:

"If I tell you, 'The lion was killed by the tiger,' which animal is dead?"

"If I tell you, 'The lion was killed by the tiger,' which animal killed the other one?"

"If I tell you, 'The boy was slapped by the girl,' which one slapped the other? Which one felt the slap?"

"If I tell you, 'The car was damaged by the motorcycle,' which vehicle needs repair?"

If the patient is unable to produce the necessary one-word answers, the administration may be adapted to "yes-no" form. Thus, in the first item the examiner may ask, "Does this mean the lion is dead?" or "Does this mean the lion did the killing?"

## Comprehension of Possessive Relationship

One of the most difficult tasks for some patients is the comprehension of the relationship between two nouns that is symbolized by the possessive "s." This difficulty is highlighted when the semantic structure does not contribute to the interpretation. That is, "my sister's hat" is a semantically nonreversible relationship, which is understandable even without the "s." When both nouns are humans, however, as in "my sister's father," the weight of the discrimination falls entirely on the word order. Thus, in order to test this feature, we present the following task to the patient:

"Suppose I point to someone across the street (examiner points) and say 'That person is my wife's brother.' Am I looking at a man or a woman?" (Or, "Is that person a man? . . . Is it a woman?")

Repeat this procedure for "my sister's husband," "my uncle's daughter," "my son's wife."

An alternative test item is "Suppose I see a mother cat and a baby kitten on the floor and I pick up the kitten's mother. Did I pick up the big one or the little one?"

## Subject of Verb Complement

Verbs like "promise" and "ask" may take superficially similar syntactic structures in verb complement phrases, but imply different referents as subject of the verb complement. This is a fairly difficult syntactic comprehension test, and it may be examined with the following items:

"John asked his father to mail the letter, and he did. Who mailed the letter?"
"Susan promised her mother to bake some brownies and she did. Who baked the brownies?"

## PSYCHOLINGUISTIC EXPLORATION OF EXPRESSION

The breakdown of grammatical performance in aphasia is manifested chiefly by the unavailability of syntactic constructions, apart from the simplest and most stereotyped. At severe levels, articles, auxiliary verbs, prepositions, and inflectional endings are lost, espeially those that occur as the first, unstressed word in a sentence. Attempts to probe for these difficulties by means of structured tasks sometimes lead to performances that are at odds with spontaneous production. That is, a patient whose spontaneous speech is agrammatic may repeat short sentences of all types well, while a grammatically fluent patient may do poorly under repetition. Therefore, these formal tasks should be considered in their own right and compared with the impression gained by listening to free conversation.

Both repetition and sentence-manipulation tasks are used, since these structured test procedures permit exploring for competence with forms that may not have occurred in free conversation. Included in the sentence-repetition tasks are constructions with a preponderance of "small grammatical words," since these have proven empirically very difficult for patients with "conduction aphasia," a selective disorder of repetition.

## Repetition Tasks

Contrast between Indicative and Interrogative.

1. The man works here.
2. Does the man work here?
3. He can swim a mile.
4. Can he swim a mile?
5. He is very rich.
6. Is he very rich?
7. He sells cars
8. Does he sell cars?
9. She ought to go.
10. Ought she to go?

Conditional Construction.

1. If she cries, feed her.
2. If he moves, shoot.
3. If it rains, stay home.
4. Feed her if she cries.

5. Shoot if he moves.
6. Stay home if it rains.

## Manipulation of Verb Tense

The agrammatic patient works with a reduced repertory of verbal endings, often having only the verb stem and the "-ing" form at his disposal. Free conversation sometimes fails to give a complete sampling of his abilities with tenses, as there may be little or no reference to past or future events. Consequently, sentence-completion tests along the lines of the following are useful to find out if the patient can adjust the verb tense to past and future, following the semantic demands of the sentence.

"The baby cries every night. She did the same last night.
Last night, the baby (what?)."
"John swims every Sunday. Next Sunday, he will do the same.
Next Sunday, he (what?)."
"I work every evening and tomorrow I will do the same.
Tomorrow night, I (what?)."

## Asking Questions

"YES"-"NO" QUESTIONS. These questions begin with an initial unstressed auxiliary verb, either a form of "do" or a modal ("can," "may") followed by the subject and principal verb. This task is extremely difficult for the Broca's aphasic but is usually performed easily by Wernicke's aphasics.

"How would you ask me if it's raining?"
"How would you ask me if I have the time?"
"How would you ask a jeweler if he fixes clocks?"
"How would you ask a stranger if he speaks English?"
"How would you ask a little boy if he can write his name?"

"WH"-QUESTIONS. These are questions opening with interrogative pronouns or adverbs, such as, "who," "where," "how," "what," and "why." While the initial word is always followed by an inversion of the subject-verb sequence, this form of question is easier than the "yes"-"no" form, perhaps because it begins with a stressed word. To elicit questions in this form, the following stimuli may be used:

"How would you ask me what the weather is like outside?"
"How would you ask me the time?"
"How would you ask a salesman the price of a certain hat?"
"How would you ask where the bus stops?"
"How would you ask to find out the owner of a certain car?"

## Repetition Tasks for Conduction Aphasia

The characteristic features of this disorder, aside from difficulty with the repetition of small grammatical words, is the predominance of literal paraphasia (transposition and substitution of phonemes) in all but number words. In the case of numbers, the errors take the form of verbal paraphasia (substitution of other numbers).

REPETITION OF DIFFICULT WORDS.
Baseball player
Peanut butter
Pussy willow
Methodist Episcopal
REPETITION WITH GRAMMATICAL WORDS.
One would have been enough.
He asked where he was when we were there.
No ifs, ands, or buts.*
REPETITION OF NUMBERS AND NUMBER-WORD COMBINATIONS. (Note contrast between verbal paraphasias on numbers and literal paraphasias on non-number words.)
Fifty-seven
Eight forty-six
Forty-eight divided by sixteen
Three-quarters equals seventy-five percent

## TESTS FOR DISCONNECTION SYNDROMES
### Dissociation of Modalities in Naming

Confrontation naming is almost always at the same level of adequacy, regardless of whether the object is presented visually, by touch, or by producing its characteristic

*This item, introduced by Dr. Norman Geschwind, has almost invariably baffled conduction aphasics.

sound. Rare exceptions to this rule are found, and these exceptions are likely to involve the interruption of fibers bringing sensory information from the right cerebral hemisphere to the left, where they must be received in order to activate a verbal response.

### Naming by Touch in Either Hand

Use a collection of small objects (coin, pencil, key, eyeglasses, comb, paper clip, ring). Subject is required to keep his eyes shut, while each object is presented to the left hand to be palpated and named. In a different sequence, they are presented to the right hand for naming. If there is variability of success, repeat the series in random order of presentation until it is clear whether or not one hand is superior to the other. Clear inferiority of the left hand raises the presumption that there is an interruption of the sensory information from the right hemisphere on its way to the left, where it must be received in order to activate a verbal response. Such an interruption involves fibers going through the corpus callosum. Tactile naming may be affected by loss of touch and position sense, i.e., a primary sensory defect. Such a primary sensory defect is established if the patient fails to match objects tactually with his left hand (using multiple-choice presentation).

### Minor Hand Agraphia

Just as incoming sensory information from the minor hemisphere may be disconnected from the language system, a similar disconnection may prevent the outflow of language-related motor instructions necessary for writing with the nonpreferred hand. A disorder of this nature can be inferred only if writing is retained to at least a moderate degree in the preferred hand. If the right hand is paralyzed, reading and oral spelling may be used as a test of the functioning of the written language system. If these functions are intact,

then agraphia of the minor hand would again signify failure of transmission of linguistically organized motor instructions across the corpus callosum.

### EXTENDED NAMING VOCABULARY—THE BOSTON NAMING TEST

Since the Visual Confrontation Naming subtest contains only six items in each of six categories, many of them being easy high-frequency words, it is valuable to supplement it with a more extensive object naming test. The Boston Naming Test is a 60-item test of line-drawn objects of graded difficulty from "bed" to "abacus." The pictures have been selected so as to eliminate items that have alternative acceptable names. In the administration of this test, the subject is provided with the initial sound (phonemic cue) if he is unable to name correctly without help. Rate of success with phonemic cues is counted separately but not included in the count of items correct.

When the test is used with aphasic patients, it is discontinued after six successive failures if the patient shows evidence of discomfort or frustration. It may be continued until the end in spite of wrong responses, if the patient is responding paraphasically and is not aware of his errors or is not disturbed by them.

The Boston Naming Test correlates with the Aphasia Severity Rating ($r = .62$), with Visual Confrontation Naming (.81), Responsive Naming (.71), and with the Finger Naming subsection of the Spatial-Quantitative battery (.78). It does not correlate with the WAIS Verbal IQ (.27), nor with the Vocabulary subtest of the WAIS (.46). Correlations in the .60s are observed with the Oral Word Reading and Oral Sentence Reading tasks. Other correlations with BDAE subtests are relatively low.

The Boston Naming Test is particularly useful for detecting relatively mild word-retrieval problems, as in cases of dementia or in cases of children with developmental reading or speech problems.

Norms based on limited samples are presented in Table 9.

**Table 9.** **Scores on Boston Naming Test (60 Items) Obtained by Children, Normal Adults, and Aphasics**

| a. 30 Normal Children, Ages 5.5 to 10.5 | | | | | |
|---|---|---|---|---|---|
| Grade | Mean Age | N | Mean | SD | Range |
| Kindergarten | 5.5 | 5 | 29.6 | 5.78 | 20–37 |
| 1 | 6.5 | 5 | 29.0 | 5.55 | 20–34 |
| 2 | 7.5 | 5 | 37.0 | 4.15 | 34–45 |
| 3 | 8.5 | 5 | 38.4 | 2.94 | 33–41 |
| 4 | 9.5 | 5 | 41.6 | 3.56 | 37–47 |
| 5 | 10.5 | 5 | 43.2 | 4.07 | 37–48 |

| b. 84 Normal Adults, Ages 18 to 59 | | | | |
|---|---|---|---|---|
| | N | Mean | SD | Range |
| Breakdown by SCHOOLING: | | | | |
| 12 years or less | 15 | 55.73 | 4.42 | 42–59 |
| More than 12 years | 31 | 55.71 | 3.33 | 46–60 |
| Breakdown by AGE: | | | | |
| 18 | 1 | 42.00 | 0.00 | — |
| 20–29 | 28 | 55.86 | 2.86 | 46–60 |
| 30–39 | 23 | 56.65 | 2.84 | 47–60 |
| 40–49 | 10 | 54.40 | 3.47 | 50–60 |
| 50–59 | 22 | 55.82 | 2.63 | 49–59 |

| c. 82 Aphasics | | | | |
|---|---|---|---|---|
| Severity Level | N | Mean | SD | Range |
| 0 | 7 | 0.0 | 0.0 | 0 |
| 1 | 35 | 1.4 | 5.7 | 0–30 |
| 2 | 12 | 18.5 | 18.9 | 0–54 |
| 3 | 13 | 34.2 | 14.3 | 1–54 |
| 4 | 9 | 49.9 | 9.6 | 33–58 |
| 5 | 6 | 39.5 | 21.3 | 2–58 |

# CHAPTER 6

## *Supplementary Nonlanguage Tests*

The study of defects associated with aphasia has identified a number of higher perceptual-motor performances that are not strictly within the sphere of language, but that, like language, are vulnerable to injuries lateralized on one side or the other and, in some cases, highly localizable within a hemisphere. This section presents an examination procedure for spatial-quantitative tasks, consisting of tests for "constructional apraxia," finger agnosia, acalculia, and right-left confusion. Normative data for aphasic patients and normal adults are presented in Table 10. In addition, we present an apraxia examination covering buccofacial praxis, limb praxis, whole body movements, and serial actions with objects. The latter examination is evaluated clinically by the examiner, rather than with reference to statistical norms, which are lacking.

There are other localizing specific deficits not covered by these test procedures. A partial list would include visual agnosia, auditory agnosia, agnosia for faces (prosopagnosia), and the minor hemisphere symptoms of left-sided neglect of personal and extrapersonal space and dressing apraxia. For discussion of these disorders, refer to relevant chapters in Heilman and Valenstein (1979).

## THE SPATIAL QUANTITATIVE BATTERY

### Constructional Deficits

Deficits in the execution of visuospatial tasks, as in drawing, assembling stick designs, and constructing three-dimensional block arrangements are commmonly referred to as "constructional apraxia." Constructional abilities are somewhat vulnerable to injuries in any part of the cortex, but the most severe disorganization of these efforts is associated with lesions encompassing both frontal and parietal lobes. While either left- or right-sided damage may produce severe deficits in construction, the most dramatic errors occur with right parietal damage, and total failure is common with bilateral parietal lobe damage.

**Table 10. Mean, Standard Deviation, and Range of Aphasics on Subtests of the Spatial-Quantitative Battery**

| Subtests | N | Mean | SD | Range |
|---|---|---|---|---|
| Draw to Command | 227 | 6.1 | 3.8 | 0–13 |
| Draw to Copy | 179 | 9.5 | 3.2 | 0–13 |
| Sticks (Memory) | 223 | 7.7 | 3.7 | 0–14 |
| Sticks (Copy) | 194 | 12.5 | 2.5 | 0–14 |
| Fingers (Total) | 214 | 97.9 | 34.8 | 0–152 |
| Fingers (Comprehension) | 190 | 32.3 | 14.2 | 0–48 |
| Fingers (Naming) | 176 | 11.6 | 11.7 | 0–32 |
| Fingers (Paired to Picture) | 176 | 17.8 | 4.2 | 0–20 |
| Fingers (Two-Finger Positions) | 188 | 17.9 | 3.5 | 0–20 |
| Fingers (Tactile) | 169 | 22.6 | 5.3 | 0–32 |
| Right-Left Orientation | 218 | 8.2 | 4.9 | 0–16 |
| Arithmetic (Total) | 228 | 11.8 | 9.5 | 0–32 |
| 3-D Blocks (Photo) | 197 | 5.9 | 3.3 | 0–10 |
| 3-D Blocks (Model) | 140 | 8.6 | 2.5 | 0–10 |
| Map Orientation | 217 | 9.4 | 4.7 | 0–14 |
| Clocks | 222 | 6.6 | 3.7 | 0–12 |

Constructional difficulties in this battery are sampled by three subtests:
  Drawing to Command
  Stick Construction (Memory)
  Three-Dimensional Blocks

DRAWING TO COMMAND. The patient is required to draw each of the following to command on a blank sheet of paper, receiving up to 3 points of credit on the first item and up to 2 points on the remaining 5, for a total possible score of 13.

This subtest correlates best with 3-D Block Construction (.61) and next best with Stick Construction Memory (.60).

*Clock*
Instruction: "Draw the *face of a clock* showing the numbers and the two hands, set to ten after eleven."
  Score: 0 to 3. One point each for:
  Approximately circular face
  Symmetry of number placement
  Correctness of numbers
  (The correctness of the setting of the hands is not scored, but provides valuable qualitative information.)

*Daisy*
Instruction: "Draw a *daisy*."
  Score: 0 to 2. One point each for:
  General shape—center with petals around it
  Symmetry of petal arrangement

*Elephant*
Instruction: "Draw an *elephant*."
  Score: 0 to 2. One point each for:
  General shape (legs, trunk, head, body)
  Relative proportions correct

*Cross*
Instruction: "You know what the *Red Cross* looks like? Draw an outline of it without taking your pencil off the paper."
  Score: 0 to 2. One point each for:
  Basic configuration
  Ability to form all corners adequately with a continuous line

*Cube*
Instructions: "Draw a *cube-shaped block* in perspective, as it would look if you could see the top and two sides."
  Score: 0 to 2. One point each for:

Grossly correct attempt
Correctness of perspective

*House*
Instruction: "Draw a *house* in perspective, so you can see the roof and two sides."
  Score: 0 to 2. One point each for:
  Grossly correct features of house
  Accuracy of perspective

Models for copying each of these should then be provided by the examiner (Figure 5a). It is of interest to see if copying is much better than drawing to command without a model. Drawing to command and drawing from a model were strongly correlated (.78).

STICK CONSTRUCTION MEMORY. Matchstick geometric figures have long been used in informal clinical tests of constructional ability. They are discussed by Goldstein and Scheerer (1941), who also published a test using plastic sticks. The present version differs in two ways from the Goldstein-Scheerer test. First, it is shorter and graduated more steeply in difficulty, to tap the normal range of ability. Secondly, while three items (W- and Z-shaped figures, and house-shaped figure) may be encoded in memory as a familiar unit (= Goldstein's "concrete"), our interest was not in contrasting codable vs. noncodable, but in scaling constructional ability.

The materials consist of 14 wooden sticks ¼-inch square by 3 inches long, 7 for the examiner's demonstrations and 7 for the patient.

Each of the 14 designs in Figure 5b is first assembled before the patient by the examiner, who instructs the patient to watch closely, since he will be expected to make the same designs. After the design has been exposed for 10 seconds, it is swept up, and the patient is given the signal to reproduce it.

Scoring is based on one point per correct item. Every stick must be in its position for credit to be allowed, although minor inaccuracies in the size of angles need not be penalized.

THREE-DIMENSIONAL BLOCKS. Three-dimensional block construction has moderately strong intercorrelations with other subtests within the spatial-quantitative cluster. The highest are with Sticks (.63), and Drawing to Command (.61). There are no correlations

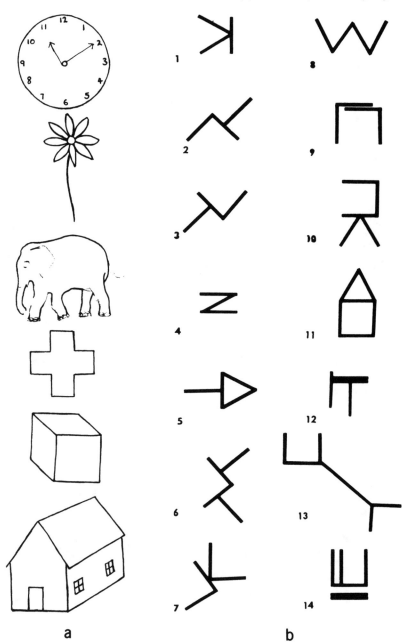

**Fig. 5.** a, Models for drawing; b, Stick test figures.

over .40 with oral language subtests, and scattered correlations in the .40s with written language tests.

The materials consist of miniature kindergarten blocks. The dimensions of the blocks and the photographs of the ten three-dimensional constructions presented for the patient to reproduce, appear in Figure 6. Time is recorded for each construction and complete accuracy of placement is required for credit—one point per item.

## Finger Agnosia

Finger recognition is performed with few or no errors by normal adults. Its impairment was identified by Gerstmann (1940) as a component, along with right-left disorientation, agraphia, and acalculia, of a syndrome associated with a lesion of the major parietal lobe, specifically of the angular gyrus. For this reason, the set of spatial and computational tests were referred to as a Parietal Lobe Battery in

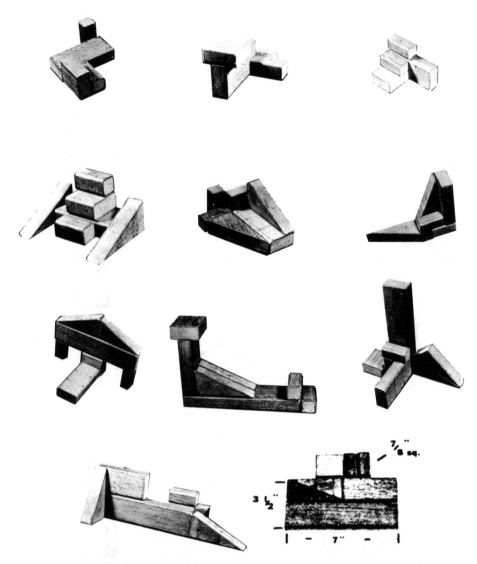

**Fig. 6.**    Three-dimensional block designs (dimensions of blocks are multiples of ⅞ inch = thickness of blocks).

the 1972 edition. Subsequent experience with these tasks has failed to support the notion that parietal lobe injury alone, in aphasics, produces selective impairment of these functions. Performance is depressed in aphasics with a lesion bridging both frontal and parietal lobes. These data do not dispute the existence of Gerstmann's syndrome as a focal feature in patients who are only mildly aphasic or otherwise intellectually unimpaired. Localizing significance should be attributed to finger identification problems, however, only when they are outstandingly severe in comparison with deficits in oral language, and

when they are accompanied by at least two of the other elements of Gerstmann's syndrome. The examiner should bear in mind these cautions in interpreting the finger identification test. Correlations in the present sample between picture identification tasks and other spatial and computational tests were low, generally below .40, as were their correlations with the verbal subtests. Finger Identification to auditory command and Finger Naming, however, were highly correlated with the most similar verbal subtests (e.g., .77 correlation between Finger Naming and Confrontation

Naming; .72 correlation between Finger Comprehension and Word Discrimination.)

Materials consist of drawings of a left and a right hand, palm down, and a hand-shielding box (Figure 7), which are used for the visual-tactile matching subset.

Prior to testing, rings are removed from patient's fingers, in order to eliminate cues as to the "ring finger," and the examiner reviews the standard names: "thumb," "index," "middle," "ring," and "little" finger. Because of the greater sensitivity to confusion found among the middle three fingers, the following weighting of scores is applied in all subsections of the test: three middle fingers—two points each; thumb and little finger—one point each.

VERBAL.

1. *Comprehension.*

   a. *Picture Hand.*

   TRIAL A. Place drawing with fingers oriented to patient. Instruct patient to indicate which finger you name. If no errors are made, allow full credit on Trial B and on Part b—own hand. Each finger is sampled twice, randomizing order of presentation.

   TRIAL B. (Omit with credit if Trial A is perfect.) Place drawing with fingers oriented away from patient and proceed as in Trial A. Score for each trial, 0 to 16.

   b. *Own Hand.*

   (Omit and credit if either Trial A or Trial B is perfectly performed.) Examiner names and patient indicates corresponding finger of either hand. Same sequence and scoring as in preceding tests.

2. *Finger Naming* (using picture).

   TRIAL A. Picture oriented with fingers toward patient. Each finger is pointed to twice in random order for patient to name, with a total possible score of 16. Omit Trial B with full credit if no errors are made on Trial A.

   TRIAL B. Same as Trial A, with fingers oriented away from patient.

   VISUAL-VISUAL.

1. *Paired-Finger Identification.* Patient's left (or nonhemiplegic) hand is placed on table, and picture of hand is oriented at right angles to it. Patient is instructed to move or point to the two fingers of his hand corresponding to those that examiner touches simultaneously on the drawing.

   Score: Allow two points per item; no partial credit.

   Sequence for paired-finger identification:

| | |
|---|---|
| thumb-little _____ | thumb-index _____ |
| middle-ring _____ | ring-little _____ |
| index-little _____ | index-middle _____ |
| thumb-middle _____ | thumb-ring _____ |
| index-ring _____ | middle-little _____ |
| | Subscore (0–20) _____ |

2. *Matching Two-Finger Positions.* Examiner holds up pairs of fingers, dorsal side to patient, asking patient to copy the gesture with the same fingers. Follow the same sequence as in paired-finger identification.

TACTILE-VISUAL. Patient inserts hand into box-shield, on upper surface of which is placed the picture of the hand corresponding to the hand being tested. Examiner touches each finger twice in random order, and patient points it out on the picture. Each hand should be tested unless there is no tactile sensation in one hand. Using a scoring system of 2 points for the 3 middle fingers and 1 point for the thumb and little fingers, the maximum score for both hands is 32. (Box-shield is illustrated in Figure 7.)

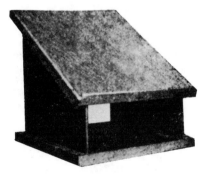

**Fig. 7.** Box-shield used for tactile-visual finger matching.

SUMMARY OF POSSIBLE SCORES.

*Verbal*
1. Comprehension
    a. Picture Hand                                0–32
    b. Own Hand                                    0–16
2. Finger Naming                                   0–32

    Subtotal                    80

*Visual-Visual*
1. Paired-Finger Identification           0–20
2. Matching Two-Finger Positions   0–20

    Subtotal                    40

*Tactile-Visual*                                    0–32

    Subtotal                    32
    Total Possible          152

## Acalculia

Disturbances of calculation are not exclusive to parietal lobe injury. The memory and mental manipulations that are required suffer from brain damage of many types. Very severe loss of number sense and of the principles of arithmetic operations (especially when reinforced by deficits in finger recognition and right-left orientation), however, are more indicative of selective parietal lesions than is a general lowering of scores.

When the patient confuses the columns in addition or subtraction, but preserves the individual numeric operations, one may suspect the spatial confusion associated with *right* parietal damage. Aphasic patients may mis-

name numbers as they write them. In some cases, they go on to a correct written solution in spite of their paraphasic sidetalk but, in some cases, they are diverted by their misnaming and carry out operations on the erroneously spoken numbers.

ARITHMETIC. Within the spatial-quantitative cluster, the arithmetic subtest correlates best with 3-D Blocks (.58), Total Fingers (.58), and Right-Left Orientation (.62). Arithmetic also has strong correlations with Serial Writing (.75) and Written Naming (.72), however, as well as with a number of reading and auditory comprehension subtests.

The following items of progressive complexity are given for solution with paper and pencil.

*Addition*

| 3 | 11 | 14 | 16 | 12 | 96 | 589 | 273 |
|---|---|---|---|---|---|---|---|
| +5 | + 8 | +13 | +27 | 45 | 53 | 234 | 491 |
| | | | | +32 | 28 | + 163 | 587 |
| | | | | | +17 | | +169 |

*Subtraction*

| 8 | 17 | 16 | 29 | 52 | 549 | 352 | 500 |
|---|---|---|---|---|---|---|---|
| −5 | − 4 | − 8 | − 16 | −25 | −138 | − 269 | − 349 |

*Multiplication*

| 2 × 3 = | 3 × 6 = | 8 × 7 = | 12 | 23 | 214 | 358 |
|---|---|---|---|---|---|---|
| | | | × 3 | ×12 | × 35 | ×679 |

Division

$$2\sqrt{6} \qquad 4\sqrt{16} \qquad 8\sqrt{168} \qquad 7\sqrt{434} \qquad 9\sqrt{621} \qquad 25\sqrt{150}$$

$$14\sqrt{161} \qquad\qquad 68\sqrt{22100} \qquad\qquad 489\sqrt{27384}$$

Answers

| Addition | Subtraction | Multiplication | Division |
|---|---|---|---|
| 8 | 3 | 6 | 3 |
| 19 | 13 | 18 | 4 |
| 27 | 8 | 56 | 21 |
| 43 | 13 | 36 | 62 |
| 89 | 27 | 276 | 69 |
| 194 | 411 | 7,490 | 6 |
| 986 | 83 | 243,082 | 11½ |
| 1,520 | 151 | | 325 |
| | | | 56 |

One point each, score: 0–32

CLOCK SETTING. While clock setting logically entails a sense of number relations, it also brings into play geometric representation. On both counts it is sensitive to spatial-quantitative impairments. In our sample, Clock Setting correlated as highly with Serial Writing (.60) and with Word Discrimination (.54) as with subtests of the spatial-quantitative cluster. Within the latter group, it is correlated with 3-D Blocks (.51), Stick Construction (.55), and Arithmetic (.64).

Clock Setting is administered by showing the patient a sheet on which four blank clock faces are drawn, with only short lines marking the positions of the 12 numbers. The patient is asked to draw in the two hands of the clock to make the faces read 1:00, 3:00, 9:15, and 7:30. Scoring is based on one point for the correct placement of each hand plus one point for indicating correctly the relative lengths of the hour and minute hands, allowing three points per item and a 0-to-12 point range for this subtest.

## Right-Left Orientation

Right-Left Orientation is one of the four components of Gerstmann's syndrome, along with finger agnosia, calculation disorder, and agraphia. In the spatial-quantitative cluster, Right-Left Orientation correlates best with Arithmetic (.62) and Finger Total (.67). It has a number of strong correlations with writing tasks, notably Primer-Level Dictation (.68), Serial Writing (.59), and correlations in the .50s with auditory and reading tasks on the one-word level.

The following commands are presented, with the most difficult given first and, if passed, credit allowed for all remaining items. If the first two items of any group are failed, skip to the next easier level. Score one point for a correct response. The maximum score is 16.

*Double-Other Person.*
(Crossed)* Point with your right hand to my right shoulder.
(Uncrossed) Point with your left hand to my right eye.
(Crossed) Point with your left hand to my left hand.
(Uncrossed) Point with your right hand to my left ear.

---

*Requires patient to cross the midline of his body.

*Double-Own Body.*
(Crossed) Put your left hand on your right ear.
(Uncrossed) Put your right hand on your right eye.
(Crossed) Put your right hand on your left shoulder.
(Uncrossed) Put your left hand on your left ear.

*Single-Other Person.*
Show me my right hand.
Show me my left shoulder.
Show me my left ear.
Show me my right eye.

*Single-Self.*
Show me your right hand.
Show me your left eye.
Show me your left shoulder.
Show me your right ear.

Since the test is given orally, allowance must be made for auditory comprehension difficulty of aphasic patients. In order to be considered significantly depressed, the percentile value for Right-Left Orientation should be lower than that for the Body-Part Identification subtest.

## APRAXIA

Apraxia refers to the loss of capacity to carry out purposeful movements, when motor strength and coordination are adequate. When apraxia is severe, it takes the form of ineptness in manipulating everyday objects. More often, it is milder, and is expressed in the inability to carry out pretended movements on request. Having an actual object in hand is a cue for normal motor behavior in using it.

The hierarchic order of difficulty between pretended actions to command and those determined by concrete contextual cues is observed in most cases, with performance to imitation lying between them in difficulty. It is not clear, however, whether this sequence of difficulty is universal.

Apraxia may affect movements of the face and buccorespiratory apparatus, autonomously from limb movements. Limb apraxia is commonly bilateral, although paralysis of one side may obscure it. Except for "dressing apraxia," these movement disorders are overwhelmingly associated with lesions of the left hemisphere and therefore are commonly associated with aphasia. There does not appear to be a psychologic causal relationship between apraxia and aphasia, however, since they vary independently as to presence and severity. The lesions of apraxia generally lie within the same gross brain areas as those causing aphasia. The precise relation between apractic symptom and lesion localization has not been as well established as the corresponding relationships for language disturbance. For a proposed theory of localization, the reader is referred to Geschwind (1975).

For the examination outlined subsequently, there are as yet no norms. Previous experience (Goodglass and Kaplan, 1963) shows that raters agree well on judgments of "normal," "partially adequate," and "failed."

The following are features of particular interest.

### Body Part As Object (BPO)

Apraxic patients have a strong tendency to represent the use of an implement by making the hand or finger take the role of the implement and come into contact with the object of the action. Thus, the index finger rubbed against the teeth becomes the toothbrush in response to, "Show me how you would pretend to brush your teeth with a toothbrush." The fist pounded on a surface becomes the hammer in response to, "Show me how you would pretend to hammer a nail."

This behavior is the rule up to 8 years of age (Kaplan, 1968), but is quite rare in normal adults. When a patient performs in this way, he should be instructed to try again as though he were really holding the implement in his hand. If this does not modify the performance, the examiner demonstrates and invites the patient to imitate. The ability to correct performance on verbal instructions is counterindicative of apraxia, while the inability to change even after demonstration is typical of the apraxic patient.

### Verbalizing Instead of Performing Buccal Commands

Patients with buccofacial apraxia, in response to instructions to "cough" or "blow," sometimes explosively utter the name of the action in their effort to carry it out, even repeating this performance after demonstration by the examiner. This occurs only with performances that require the activation of the oral-respiratory apparatus.

## Whole-Body (Axial) Commands

Several commands requiring actions that involve the body axis are included in the examination. These commands are of particular interest in patients with severe auditory comprehension disorders, since many commands of this type are well performed by patients who do not understand limb commands. Geschwind (1975) points out that axial movements are innervated by bilateral, nonpyramidal motor tracts, unlike limb movements, which appear to be dependent on left hemisphere engrams and, consequently, on left hemisphere language.

### Apraxia Test

| Movements to Oral Command | Movements to Imitation | Movements with Real Object |
|---|---|---|
| *Buccofacial* | | |
| 1. Cough | If failed to command | Does not apply |
| 2. Sniff | If failed to command | If failed to command |
| 3. Blow out a match | If failed to command | If failed to command |
| 4. Suck through a straw | If failed to command | If failed to command |
| 5. Puff out cheeks | If failed to command | Does not apply |
| *Intransitive Limb* | | |
| 1. Wave good-bye | If failed to command | Does not apply |
| 2. Beckon "come here" | If failed to command | Does not apply |
| 3. Finger on lip for "shsh" | If failed to command | Does not apply |
| 4. Salute | If failed to command | Does not apply |
| 5. Signal "stop" | If failed to command | Does not apply |
| *Transitive Limb* | | |
| 1. Brush teeth | If failed to command | If failed to command |
| 2. Stir coffee with a spoon | If failed to command | If failed to command |
| 3. Hammer | If failed to command | If failed to command |
| 4. Saw board | If failed to command | If failed to command |
| 5. Use screwdriver | If failed to command | If failed to command |
| *Whole Body* | | |
| 1. How does a boxer stand? | If failed to command | Does not apply |
| 2. How does a golfer stand? | If failed to command | Does not apply |
| 3. How does a soldier march in place? | If failed to command | Does not apply |
| 4. How do you shovel snow? | If failed to command | Does not apply |
| 5. Stand up, turn around twice, and sit down. | If failed to command | Does not apply |

*Serial Actions* (with real objects only)
1. Provide box of matches and pack of cigarettes.
   "Take a cigarette and light up."
2. Provide paper, envelope, and stamp.
   "Put the paper in the envelope, seal it, and stamp it."
3. Provide candle, candlestick, box of matches.
   "Put the candle in the holder, light it, and blow it out."

## PERFORMANCE OF NORMAL SUBJECTS

Borod, Goodglass, and Kaplan (1980) obtained normative data on the subtests of the Spatial-Quantitative battery from 147 neurologically normal adult males, ages 25 to 85, and ranging in education from less than 8 grades through college. As compared to the uniformly high scores obtained by normal subjects in the language subtests, scores on these tasks are considerably wider in range and more clearly related to age and education. We therefore reproduce in Table 11 the data stratified both by age and by education. It should be noted that age and education are confounded in that the lowest education group is largely composed of elderly subjects.

**Table 11. Scores Attained by Normal Adults on Subtests of the Spatial-Quantitative Battery***

*Drawings to Command*

| Age | Signif. | N | X̄ | SD | Lowest Score | First Quartile | Second Quartile | Third Quartile | Highest Score |
|---|---|---|---|---|---|---|---|---|---|
| under 40 | | 38 | 11.5 | 1.8 | | 7 | 11 | 12 | 13 | 13 |
| 40–49 | | 17 | 10.5 | 2.6 | | 5 | 10 | 11 | 13 | 13 |
| 50–59 | | 33 | 10.6 | 1.7 | | 7 | 10 | 11 | 12 | 13 |
| 60–69 | | 30 | 9.7 | 2.0 | | 6 | 8 | 10 | 11 | 12 |
| 70 and over | | 27 | 9.5 | 2.7 | | 4 | 9 | 10 | 11 | 13 |
| Total | | 145 | 10.4 | 2.2 | | | | | | |
| Education | | | | | | | | | |
| 0–8 years | | 9 | 8.0 | 2.1 | | 4 | 6 | 9 | 10 | 10 |
| 9–12 years | | 67 | 10.1 | 2.5 | | 8 | 9 | 11 | 12 | 13 |
| 13–16 years | | 56 | 11.0 | 1.9 | | 7 | 10 | 11 | 13 | 13 |
| Total | | 132 | 10.4 | 2.2 | | | | | | |

*Drawings to Copy*

| Age | Signif. | N | X̄ | SD | Lowest Score | First Quartile | Second Quartile | Third Quartile | Highest Score |
|---|---|---|---|---|---|---|---|---|---|
| under 40 | | 37 | 12.4 | 1.0 | | 10 | 12 | 13 | 13 | 13 |
| 40–49 | | 16 | 11.8 | 1.6 | | 7 | 11 | 12 | 13 | 13 |
| 50–59 | | 31 | 12.4 | 1.0 | | 10 | 12 | 13 | 13 | 13 |
| 60–69 | | 29 | 11.7 | 1.1 | | 8 | 11 | 12 | 12.8 | 13 |
| 70 and over | | 25 | 11.2 | 2.0 | | 6 | 11 | 11.5 | 13 | 13 |
| Total | | 138 | 12.2 | 1.4 | | | | | | |
| Education | | | | | | | | | |
| 0–8 years | | 8 | 10.3 | 2.2 | | 7 | 7 | 11 | 12 | 13 |
| 9–12 years | | 62 | 11.7 | 1.5 | | 6 | 11 | 12 | 13 | 13 |
| 13–16 years | | 55 | 12.2 | 1.0 | | 10 | 11 | 13 | 13 | 13 |
| Total | | 125 | 11.9 | 1.5 | | | | | | |

*Bracketing across groups in "Signif." column indicates that means for these groups do not differ at the .05 level.

*Sticks to Memory*

| Age | Signif. | N | $\bar{X}$ | SD | | Lowest Score | First Quartile | Second Quartile | Third Quartile | Highest Score |
|---|---|---|---|---|---|---|---|---|---|---|
| under 40 | } | 37 | 12.7 | 1.1 | | 9 | 12 | 13 | 13 | 14 |
| 40–49 | } | 17 | 12.4 | 1.9 | | 7 | 11 | 12.5 | 14 | 14 |
| 50–59 | | 30 | 11.4 | 1.7 | | 7 | 10.5 | 11 | 12.5 | 14 |
| 60–69 | | 30 | 10.6 | 2.9 | | 3 | 10 | 12 | 12 | 14 |
| 70 and over | | 27 | 9.9 | 3.7 | | 1 | 7.75 | 11 | 13 | 14 |
| | | | | | | | | | | |
| Total | | 141 | 11.4 | 2.6 | | | | | | |
| | | | | | | | | | | |
| Education | | | | | | | | | | |
| 0–8 years | } | 9 | 10.2 | 2.7 | | 4 | 8.3 | 10.5 | 12 | 13 |
| 9–12 years | } | 64 | 11.3 | 2.8 | | 1 | 10 | 12 | 13 | 14 |
| 13–16 years | | 55 | 11.4 | 2.5 | | 3 | 11 | 12 | 13 | 14 |
| | | | | | | | | | | |
| Total | | 128 | 11.2 | 2.7 | | | | | | |

*Sticks to Copy*

| Age | Signif. | N | $\bar{X}$ | SD | | Lowest Score | First Quartile | Second Quartile | Third Quartile | Highest Score |
|---|---|---|---|---|---|---|---|---|---|---|
| under 40 | } | 37 | 13.8 | .4 | | 12 | 14 | 14 | 14 | 14 |
| 40–49 | | 17 | 13.8 | .8 | | 11 | 14 | 14 | 14 | 14 |
| 50–59 | } | 30 | 13.9 | .4 | | 12 | 14 | 14 | 14 | 14 |
| 60–69 | | 30 | 13.4 | 1.5 | | 6 | 13 | 14 | 14 | 14 |
| 70 and over | | 27 | 13.3 | 1.7 | | 8 | 14 | 14 | 14 | 14 |
| | | | | | | | | | | |
| Total | | 141 | 13.6 | 1.1 | | | | | | |
| | | | | | | | | | | |
| Education | | | | | | | | | | |
| 0–8 years | } | 9 | 13.9 | .3 | | 13 | 14 | 14 | 14 | 14 |
| 9–12 years | } | 64 | 13.4 | 1.5 | | 6 | 13 | 14 | 14 | 14 |
| 13–16 years | | 55 | 13.8 | .5 | | 12 | 14 | 14 | 14 | 14 |
| | | | | | | | | | | |
| Total | | 128 | 13.6 | 1.2 | | | | | | |

*Three-Dimensional Blocks from Photographs*

| Age | Signif. | N | X̄ | SD | | Lowest Score | First Quartile | Second Quartile | Third Quartile | Highest Score |
|---|---|---|---|---|---|---|---|---|---|---|
| under 40 | | 36 | 9.5 | .9 | | 6 | 9 | 10 | 10 | 10 |
| 40–49 | | 17 | 8.8 | 1.7 | | 3 | 8 | 9 | 10 | 10 |
| 50–59 | | 29 | 8.4 | 1.6 | | 3 | 8 | 9 | 9.8 | 10 |
| 60–69 | | 29 | 7.4 | 2.8 | | 0 | 5.3 | 8 | 9.8 | 10 |
| 70 and over | | 26 | 6.8 | 2.5 | | 2 | 5 | 7 | 9 | 10 |
| | | | | | | | | | | |
| Total | | 137 | 8.2 | 2.2 | | | | | | |
| | | | | | | | | | | |
| Education | | | | | | | | | | |
| 0–8 years | | 9 | 7.4 | 2.4 | | 4 | 4.25 | 7.5 | 9.75 | 10 |
| 9–12 years | | 61 | 8.3 | 2.2 | | 2 | 7 | 9 | 10 | 10 |
| 13–16 years | | 54 | 8.1 | 2.5 | | 0 | 7 | 9 | 10 | 10 |
| | | | | | | | | | | |
| Total | | 124 | 8.1 | 2.4 | | | | | | |

*Three-Dimensional Blocks from Models*

| Age | Signif. | N | X̄ | SD | | Lowest Score | First Quartile | Second Quartile | Third Quartile | Highest Score |
|---|---|---|---|---|---|---|---|---|---|---|
| under 40 | | 37 | 9.9 | .3 | | 9 | 10 | 10 | 10 | 10 |
| 40–49 | | 16 | 10.0 | .0 | | 10 | 10 | 10 | 10 | 10 |
| 50–59 | | 27 | 9.9 | .4 | | 8 | 10 | 10 | 10 | 10 |
| 60–69 | | 30 | 9.6 | 1.7 | | 1 | 10 | 10 | 10 | 10 |
| 70 and over | | 26 | 9.4 | 1.2 | | 4 | 9 | 10 | 10 | 10 |
| | | | | | | | | | | |
| Total | | 136 | 9.7 | 1.0 | | | | | | |
| | | | | | | | | | | |
| Education | | | | | | | | | | |
| 0–8 years | | 9 | 9.7 | .5 | | 9 | 9 | 10 | 10 | 10 |
| 9–12 years | | 60 | 9.8 | .8 | | 4 | 10 | 10 | 10 | 10 |
| 13–16 years | | 54 | 9.6 | 1.3 | | 1 | 10 | 10 | 10 | 10 |
| | | | | | | | | | | |
| Total | | 123 | 9.7 | 1.1 | | | | | | |

*Total Fingers*

| Age | Signif. | N | X̄ | SD | | Lowest Score | First Quartile | Second Quartile | Third Quartile | Highest Score |
|---|---|---|---|---|---|---|---|---|---|---|
| under 40 | ⎫ | 37 | 150 | 4.5 | | 132 | 151 | 152 | 152 | 152 |
| 40–49 | ⎬ ⎫ | 17 | 149 | 4.4 | | 136 | 146 | 151 | 152 | 152 |
| 50–59 | ⎬ | 29 | 149 | 3.4 | | 136 | 148 | 149 | 152 | 152 |
| 60–69 | ⎭ | 29 | 147 | 6.3 | | 122 | 144 | 148 | 152 | 152 |
| 70 and over | ⎭ | 26 | 145 | 8.1 | | 121 | 141 | 148 | 152 | 152 |
| | | | | | | | | | | |
| Total | | 138 | 148.1 | 5.8 | | | | | | |
| | | | | | | | | | | |
| Education | | | | | | | | | | |
| 0–8 years | ⎫ | 9 | 146 | 10.3 | | 121 | 142 | 152 | 152 | 152 |
| 9–12 years | ⎬ | 62 | 148 | 4.7 | | 135 | 147 | 150 | 152 | 152 |
| 13–16 years | ⎭ | 54 | 148 | 6.5 | | 122 | 146 | 152 | 152 | 152 |
| | | | | | | | | | | |
| Total | | 125 | 147.9 | 6.0 | | | | | | |

*Fingers—Verbal*

| Age | Signif. | N | X̄ | SD | | Lowest Score | First Quartile | Second Quartile | Third Quartile | Highest Score |
|---|---|---|---|---|---|---|---|---|---|---|
| under 40 | ⎫ | 37 | 79.3 | 2.7 | | 65 | 80 | 80 | 80 | 80 |
| 40–49 | ⎬ | 17 | 79.4 | 1.5 | | 74 | 80 | 80 | 80 | 80 |
| 50–59 | ⎬ | 29 | 79.4 | .9 | | 77 | 79 | 80 | 80 | 80 |
| 60–69 | ⎬ | 29 | 77.3 | 4.6 | | 63 | 77 | 80 | 80 | 80 |
| 70 and over | ⎭ | 26 | 78.2 | 3.1 | | 68 | 77 | 80 | 80 | 80 |
| | | | | | | | | | | |
| Total | | 138 | 78.7 | 3.0 | | | | | | |
| | | | | | | | | | | |
| Education | | | | | | | | | | |
| 0–8 years | ⎫ | 9 | 79.1 | 1.4 | | 77 | 78 | 80 | 80 | 80 |
| 9–12 years | ⎬ | 62 | 78.4 | 3.3 | | 65 | 79 | 80 | 80 | 80 |
| 13–16 years | ⎭ | 54 | 79.0 | 3.0 | | 63 | 80 | 80 | 80 | 80 |
| | | | | | | | | | | |
| Total | | 125 | 78.7 | 3.1 | | | | | | |

*Fingers—Visual/Tactile*

| Age | Signif. | N | X̄ | SD | | Lowest Score | First Quartile | Second Quartile | Third Quartile | Highest Score |
|---|---|---|---|---|---|---|---|---|---|---|
| under 40 | | 37 | 70.8 | 3.5 | | 52 | 72 | 72 | 72 | 72 |
| 40–49 | | 17 | 69.2 | 4.6 | | 58 | 67 | 72 | 72 | 72 |
| 50–59 | | 29 | 69.4 | 3.1 | | 58 | 68 | 70 | 72 | 72 |
| 60–69 | | 29 | 68.0 | 4.2 | | 58 | 66 | 69 | 72 | 72 |
| 70 and over | | 26 | 66.7 | 6.0 | | 51 | 64 | 69 | 72 | 72 |
| | | | | | | | | | | |
| Total | | 138 | 68.9 | 4.5 | | | | | | |
| | | | | | | | | | | |
| Education | | | | | | | | | | |
| 0–8 years | | 9 | 67.3 | 7.4 | | 51 | 63 | 72 | 72 | 72 |
| 9–12 years | | 62 | 69.1 | 4.0 | | 56 | 68 | 71 | 72 | 72 |
| 13–16 years | | 54 | 68.8 | 4.9 | | 52 | 66 | 72 | 72 | 72 |
| | | | | | | | | | | |
| Total | | 125 | 68.8 | 4.7 | | | | | | |

*Right-Left Orientation*

| Age* | Signif. | N | X̄ | SD | | Lowest Score | First Quartile | Second Quartile | Third Quartile | Highest Score |
|---|---|---|---|---|---|---|---|---|---|---|
| under 40 | | 39 | 15.8 | .5 | | 14 | 16 | 16 | 16 | 16 |
| 40–49 | | 14 | 15.8 | .5 | | 14 | 16 | 16 | 16 | 16 |
| 50–59 | | 32 | 15.7 | .8 | | 12 | 16 | 16 | 16 | 16 |
| 60–69 | | 29 | 15.2 | 1.0 | | 13 | 14 | 16 | 16 | 16 |
| 70 and over | | 26 | 15.4 | 1.1 | | 12 | 15 | 16 | 16 | 16 |
| | | | | | | | | | | |
| Total | | 140 | 15.5 | .8 | | | | | | |
| | | | | | | | | | | |
| Education | | | | | | | | | | |
| 0–8 years | | 9 | 15.6 | .5 | | 15 | 15 | 16 | 16 | 16 |
| 9–12 years | | 63 | 15.5 | .9 | | 12 | 15 | 16 | 16 | 16 |
| 13–16 years | | 56 | 15.6 | .8 | | 12 | 16 | 16 | 16 | 16 |
| | | | | | | | | | | |
| Total | | 128 | 15.5 | .8 | | | | | | |

*The only significant difference is between subjects under 40 and those between 60 and 69.

*Clock Setting (Without Numbers)*

| Age | Signif. | N | X̄ | SD | | Lowest Score | First Quartile | Second Quartile | Third Quartile | Highest Score |
|---|---|---|---|---|---|---|---|---|---|---|
| under 40 | | 36 | 11.6 | 1.1 | | 8 | 12 | 12 | 12 | 12 |
| 40–49 | | 16 | 10.9 | 1.6 | | 8 | 10 | 12 | 12 | 12 |
| 50–59 | | 32 | 10.8 | 1.5 | | 8 | 10 | 12 | 12 | 12 |
| 60–69 | | 28 | 10.1 | 2.4 | | 2 | 9 | 11 | 12 | 12 |
| 70 and over | | 26 | 10.2 | 2.5 | | 5 | 8 | 12 | 12 | 12 |
| | | | | | | | | | | |
| Total | | 138 | 10.7 | 1.9 | | | | | | |
| | | | | | | | | | | |
| Education | | | | | | | | | | |
| 0–8 years | | 8 | 8.9 | 2.7 | | 5 | 6 | 10 | 11 | 12 |
| 9–12 years | | 63 | 10.6 | 2.0 | | 2 | 9 | 12 | 12 | 12 |
| 13–16 years | | 55 | 11.2 | 1.4 | | 8 | 11 | 12 | 12 | 12 |
| | | | | | | | | | | |
| Total | | 126 | 10.7 | 1.9 | | | | | | |

*Clock Setting (Prenumbered Face)*

| Age | Signif. | N | X̄ | SD | | Lowest Score | First Quartile | Second Quartile | Third Quartile | Highest Score |
|---|---|---|---|---|---|---|---|---|---|---|
| under 40 | | 29 | 11.7 | .7 | | 9 | 12 | 12 | 12 | 12 |
| 40–49 | | 11 | 11.1 | 1.6 | | 8 | 9.5 | 12 | 12 | 12 |
| 50–59 | | 21 | 11.0 | 1.3 | | 8 | 10 | 11.5 | 12 | 12 |
| 60–69 | | 25 | 11.0 | 1.9 | | 5 | 10.3 | 12 | 12 | 12 |
| 70 and over | | 25 | 10.9 | 1.9 | | 6 | 8.5 | 12 | 12 | 12 |
| | | | | | | | | | | |
| Total | | 111 | 11.2 | 1.5 | | | | | | |
| | | | | | | | | | | |
| Education | | | | | | | | | | |
| 0–8 years | | 8 | 10.0 | 2.2 | | 6 | 8 | 10 | 12 | 12 |
| 9–12 years | | 58 | 10.9 | 1.7 | | 5 | 10 | 12 | 12 | 12 |
| 13–16 years | | 39 | 11.6 | .9 | | 8 | 12 | 12 | 12 | 12 |
| | | | | | | | | | | |
| Total | | 105 | 11.1 | 1.6 | | | | | | |

*Total Arithmetic*

| Age | Signif. | N | X̄ | SD | | Lowest Score | First Quartile | Second Quartile | Third Quartile | Highest Score |
|---|---|---|---|---|---|---|---|---|---|---|
| under 40 | | 37 | 29.4 | 2.6 | | 19 | 28 | 30 | 31 | 32 |
| 40–49 | | 16 | 28.4 | 3.0 | | 23 | 26 | 29 | 31 | 32 |
| 50–59 | | 32 | 29.0 | 3.9 | | 15 | 28 | 30 | 31 | 32 |
| 60–69 | | 28 | 28.3 | 3.3 | | 18 | 27 | 29 | 30 | 32 |
| 70 and over | | 26 | 29.1 | 3.0 | | 20 | 27.5 | 31 | 31 | 32 |
| | | | | | | | | | | |
| Total | | 139 | 28.9 | 3.2 | | | | | | |
| | | | | | | | | | | |
| Education | | | | | | | | | | |
| 0–8 years | | 8 | 24.6 | 2.5 | | 20 | 22 | 26 | 26 | 28 |
| 9–12 years | | 63 | 28.5 | 3.7 | | 15 | 27 | 30 | 31 | 32 |
| 13–16 years | | 56 | 29.6 | 2.3 | | 19 | 28 | 30 | 31 | 32 |
| | | | | | | | | | | |
| Total | | 127 | 28.7 | 3.3 | | | | | | |

*Arithmetic—Addition and Subtraction*

| Age | Signif. | N | X̄ | SD | | Lowest Score | First Quartile | Second Quartile | Third Quartile | Highest Score |
|---|---|---|---|---|---|---|---|---|---|---|
| under 40 | | 37 | 15.2 | 1.0 | | 11 | 15 | 15 | 16 | 16 |
| 40–49 | | 16 | 15.1 | .9 | | 13 | 14 | 15 | 16 | 16 |
| 50–59 | | 32 | 15.3 | 1.2 | | 11 | 15 | 16 | 16 | 16 |
| 60–69 | | 28 | 15.1 | 1.3 | | 10 | 14 | 15 | 16 | 16 |
| 70 and over | | 26 | 15.5 | .8 | | 13 | 15 | 16 | 16 | 16 |
| | | | | | | | | | | |
| Total | | 139 | 15.2 | 1.1 | | | | | | |
| | | | | | | | | | | |
| Education | | | | | | | | | | |
| 0–8 years | | 8 | 14.4 | .9 | | 13 | 14 | 14 | 15 | 16 |
| 9–12 years | | 63 | 15.2 | 1.2 | | 10 | 15 | 16 | 16 | 16 |
| 13–16 years | | 56 | 15.3 | .9 | | 11 | 15 | 16 | 16 | 16 |
| | | | | | | | | | | |
| Total | | 127 | 15.2 | 1.1 | | | | | | |

*Arithmetic—Multiplication and Division*

| Age | Signif. | N | X̄ | SD | | Lowest Score | First Quartile | Second Quartile | Third Quartile | Highest Score |
|---|---|---|---|---|---|---|---|---|---|---|
| under 40 | ⎫ | 37 | 14.2 | 1.8 | | 8 | 13 | 14 | 16 | 16 |
| 40–49 | ⎪ | 16 | 13.3 | 2.4 | | 8 | 11 | 14 | 15 | 16 |
| 50–59 | ⎬ | 32 | 13.9 | 2.9 | | 4 | 13 | 15 | 16 | 16 |
| 60–69 | ⎪ | 28 | 13.1 | 2.4 | | 8 | 12 | 14 | 15 | 16 |
| 70 and over | ⎭ | 26 | 13.7 | 2.4 | | 7 | 12 | 15 | 15 | 16 |
| | | | | | | | | | | |
| Total | | 139 | 13.7 | 2.4 | | | | | | |
| | | | | | | | | | | |
| Education | | | | | | | | | | |
| 0–8 years | | 8 | 10.3 | 2.1 | | 7 | 7 | 11 | 12 | 12 |
| 9–12 years | ⎫⎬⎭ | 63 | 13.3 | 2.7 | | 4 | 12 | 14 | 15 | 16 |
| 13–16 years | | 56 | 14.3 | 1.6 | | 8 | 13 | 15 | 15 | 16 |
| | | | | | | | | | | |
| Total | | 127 | 13.6 | 2.5 | | | | | | |

*Map Orientation*

| Age | Signif. | N | X̄ | SD | | Lowest Score | First Quartile | Second Quartile | Third Quartile | Highest Score |
|---|---|---|---|---|---|---|---|---|---|---|
| under 40 | ⎫ | 37 | 12.8 | 1.6 | | 7 | 12 | 13 | 14 | 14 |
| 40–49 | ⎪ | 15 | 12.9 | 2.0 | | 7 | 12 | 14 | 14 | 14 |
| 50–59 | ⎬ | 30 | 12.7 | 2.8 | | 2 | 13 | 14 | 14 | 14 |
| 60–69 | ⎪ | 26 | 11.2 | 3.8 | | 0 | 11 | 13 | 14 | 14 |
| 70 and over | ⎭ | 24 | 11.2 | 3.5 | | 2 | 10 | 13 | 14 | 14 |
| | | | | | | | | | | |
| Total | | 131 | 12.2 | 2.9 | | | | | | |
| | | | | | | | | | | |
| Education | | | | | | | | | | |
| 0–8 years | | 6 | 6.5 | 4.2 | | 1 | 2 | 8 | 10 | 12 |
| 9–12 years | | 58 | 11.7 | 3.2 | | 0 | 11 | 13 | 14 | 14 |
| 13–16 years | | 54 | 13.0 | 1.8 | | 6 | 13 | 14 | 14 | 14 |
| | | | | | | | | | | |
| Total | | 118 | 12.0 | 3.5 | | | | | | |

# CHAPTER 7

# Major Aphasic Syndromes and Illustrations of Test Patterns

The various component elements in language disorders, described in detail in Chapter 2, are not free to appear in any combination or in isolation from each other. The clustering of these symptoms is in part a function of the anatomic organization of the substrate for language in the brain. Equally important in determining the makeup of the syndromes is the fact that the locations of natural lesions, particularly cerebrovascular ones, tend to congregate in certain vulnerable sites in the brain.

It has been customary in the past to emphasize differences in terminology employed by various writers in the 120-year modern history of aphasiology, as if to suggest that these differences represented profound confusion and disagreement as to the typology of the aphasias. Yet a careful reading of the clinical features that were described by Head, Goldstein, Weisenburg and McBride, Luria, Wepman, and Hécaen shows that they agreed closely on the major subtypes of aphasia and on the typical lesion sites associated with them. In most instances, the different terms they applied could be readily translated from one system to another. For such a conversion table, covering 21 writers from 1865 to 1978, see Benson (1979, pp. 60–62).

The fact that distinct configurations of language abnormality keep recurring, each in conjunction with a lesion of a different zone in the perisylvian region of the left hemisphere, is the basis for whatever knowledge we have of the anatomy of language. One must keep in mind, however, that the described syndromes represent only those symptom clusters that are seen recurrently in roughly similar form. They do not represent every case of aphasia. In fact, depending on the rigor or looseness with which the definitions are applied, estimates of the proportion of cases that can be unambiguously classified range from 30% in some centers to 80% in others. This is not surprising, nor is it discouraging as to the usefulness of the named syndromes as anchor points in our thinking about aphasia.

First, it is recognized that young children who develop aphasia from a focal lesion do not show the clearcut differentiation of symptoms that is seen in adults as a function of the lesion site. That is, the localization of symptoms with which we are familiar is the product of brain maturation and years of language use, which need not follow precisely the same path in all brains. Second, deviations from the standard association between lesion and aphasic syndrome are found in adults who develop aphasia from right-hemisphere lesions, whether they are left-handers or cases of crossed aphasia in right-handers. Specifically, the pattern of copious paraphasic speech with severely impaired comprehension has not been reported in these individuals. It appears then that variations in the lateralization of language in the brain lead to corresponding variations in the anatomic organization of the components of language.

Our present view, then, is that the syndromes that are named and described in this section represent the most regularly recurring patterns of response, in language behavior, to lesions of given sites within the language zone. Variants of these syndromes occur, not only because natural lesions vary almost infinitely in precise location and extent, but because response to the same injury is not fixed and immutable across individuals.

With the advent of the CT scan, the role of subcortical lesions in the production of aphasia has become clearly established and a number of common patterns of subcortical aphasia have been described (Benson, 1979; Alexander and LoVerme, 1980; Naeser et al., 1982). These will be reviewed later in this chapter.

## FLUENCY VS. NONFLUENCY

The major subdivision among the aphasic syndromes is based on the character of the speech output. When the prerolandic (anterior) portion of the anatomic speech area (Broca's area) is involved, the flow of speech is more or less impaired at the levels of speech initiation, finding and sequencing of articulatory movements, and production of grammatical sequences. The resulting speech—interrupted, awkwardly articulated with great effort—is referred to as "nonfluent." The contrasting or "fluent" forms of aphasia are marked by facility in articulation and many long runs of words in a variety of grammatical constructions, in conjunction with word-finding difficulty for substantives and picturable action words. The criteria for distinguishing between fluent and nonfluent aphasias are essentially those dealt with in the rating scale of speech characteristics (Chapter 4). The fluent aphasias are usually due to lesions posterior to the rolandic fissure, sparing Broca's area. Within this region, there is considerable variation in the detailed symptomatology of fluent aphasia, This variation is at least partly understandable in terms of the site of the injury. The significant variable components are the amount and type of paraphasia, auditory receptive loss, word-finding difficulty, and im-

paired repetition. The terms "fluent" and "nonfluent" are sometimes used interchangeably with "posterior" and "anterior" to characterize the major subdivisions of the aphasias.

### Broca's Aphasia

(Head—"Verbal Aphasia"; Goldstein—"Motor Aphasia"; Luria—"Efferent Motor Aphasia"; Weisenburg and McBride—"Expressive Aphasia.")

We revert to the classical eponym rather than using the term "motor" aphasia or "expressive" aphasia, in order to avoid suggesting that speech output is normal in other forms of aphasia. Broca's aphasia is the common "anterior," or "nonfluent," aphasia depending on a lesion involving the third frontal convolution of the left hemisphere, the subcortical white matter, and extending posteriorly to the inferior portion of the motor strip (precentral gyrus). Its essential characteristics are awkward articulation, restricted vocabulary, restriction of grammar to the simplest, most overlearned forms, and relative preservation of auditory comprehension. Written language follows the pattern of speech in that writing is usually impaired at least as severely as speech, while reading is only mildly affected.

At the early, severe levels, the patient may have lost even "yes" or "no" and be unable to initiate articulatory movements or to repeat any word. Nonspeech oral movements are often, *but not always,* affected. The variability of this association indicates that the articulatory failure is not caused by difficulty with oral movements per se. Comprehension of single words is prompt, but the patient may be confused by more complex spoken messages. As he begins to recover, the effortful, short-phrased quality of his speech is prominent. While a few difficult sounds may be simplified (e.g., "ts" for "ch"; "p" for "pl"), the articulatory difficulty is much reduced in imitation and may disappear in the recitation of memorized series. Thus, articulation is best judged during free conversation. Here, in addition to awkwardness and distortion of phonemes, we often hear some literal paraphasias, i.e., substitutions or transpositions of phonemes as in "pelsil" for "pencil."

At the beginning of the recovery stage, too, object-naming often returns to functional levels, while syntax remains primitive. The patient may have only one- or two-word sentences and show his maximum difficulty in combining subject and verb, so that subject-noun phrase and verb phrase are produced as separate utterances. While often the patient may try to form complete sentences, he has usually lost the ability to evoke syntactic patterns, and even a sentence repetition task may prove impossible from the grammatical point of view.

CONFIGURATION OF TEST SCORES. The Broca's aphasic, because of the sparsity and effort of his speech, is usually rated as "severe," i.e., level 1 or 2 on the severity rating scale. Level 3, however, is not uncommon as the patient continues to recover. Those Broca's aphasic patients who go on to become only mild or residual aphasics (levels 4 and 5) lose the distinctive characteristics of Broca's aphasia. Their articulation and fluency approach normal levels, and they show only some word-finding difficulty, making them barely distinguishable from mild anomic aphasics. They never show the pressure of rapid speech or the blatant circumlocution and emptiness of substantive content, however, that mark the *typical* anomic aphasic.

Figure 8 shows the range of ratings on the Profile of Speech Characteristics, consistent with Broca's aphasia.

The Aphasia Subtest Summary Profile will show the fluency and severity scores lower than the auditory comprehension and naming scores. Oral reading and repetition will tend to be on a par with severity. The paraphasia pattern might show some literal paraphasia, but little of the other varieties. Reading comprehension is typically among the highest of the score clusters, writing among the lowest.

A CASE OF BROCA'S APHASIA. J.M. was a 21-year-old, right-handed male with a tenth-grade education, wounded, 9 months prior to his examination, by a mortar shell fragment that penetrated the frontoparietal region and left him with a severe right hemiplegia and a severe Broca's aphasia. At the time of examination, he was moderately depressed but quite cooperative. During his stay in the aphasia unit, he displayed considerable artistic talent, but his poor morale prevented his following through with plans for formal art training. On a follow-up visit after 6 months at home, his speech showed essentially the same pattern described here, but with easier access to vocabulary. His spirits were greatly improved; he had become engaged to a home-town girl and made plans to enter art school.

During the initial interview his speech was limited to one-word answers, almost all nouns. The one verb used during the "cookie theft" picture narrative is uninflected, although it refers to a present progressive action. The interview required much questioning and guessing by the examiner. A sample of his production follows (E = examiner; J.M. = patient's initials):

> E.:   What did you do before you went to Vietnam?
> J.M.: Forces.
> E.:   You were in the army?
> J.M.: Special forces. (Poor articulation)
> E.:   What did you do?
> J.M.: Boom!
> E.:   I don't understand.
> J.M.: 'Splosions.
>       (Further questioning by examiner)
> J.M.: Me . . . one guy.
> E.:   Were you alone when you were injured?
> J.M.: Recon . . . scout.
> E.:   What happened; why are you here?
> J.M.: Speech.
> E.:   What happened?
> J.M.: Mortar.
>       (On presentation of "cookie theft" picture for description)
> J.M.: Cookie jar . . . fall over . . .
>       chair . . . water . . . empty . . .
>       ov . . . ov . . .
> E.:   Overflow?
> J.M.: Yeah.

The patient was rated at severity level "1," indicating that much questioning and inference were needed, with the interviewer carrying the burden of conversation.

Examination of the Subtest Summary Profile (Figure 9) shows the typical pattern for Broca's aphasics. Fluency, including articulation, is low; the severity rating is at "1," but auditory comprehension is little impaired. The naming cluster is decidedly superior to the

## RATING SCALE PROFILE OF SPEECH CHARACTERISTICS

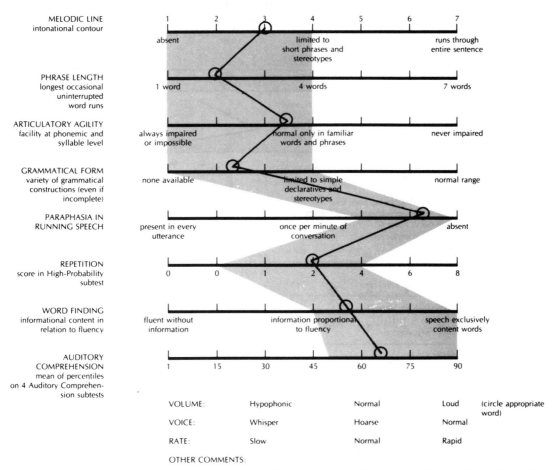

**Fig. 8.** Broca's aphasia. Shaded area indicates range of profile ratings compatible with this disorder. Heavy line indicates mean of nine representative cases. (Volume, Voice, and Rate ratings in this and following case illustrations were not available at time of examination.)

fluency level. Paraphasia is virtually absent. Reading shows only mild impairment, except for the comprehension of oral spelling. While the recall of writing movements is good, the rest of writing performance is commensurate with the patient's impaired fluency level. The spatial-quantitative cluster is at near-normal levels. A WAIS performance-scale I.Q. was 97, but when rescored without time limits, it was 127.

Examination of the Speech Characteristics Profile (Figure 10) again shows the typical Broca's aphasia pattern, with uniformly low speech melody, articulation and phrase length, absence of paraphasia, and superiority of word finding to the general fluency level. The auditory comprehension scale, based on the mean percentile of the auditory comprehension cluster, is at the near-normal level.

### Wernicke's Aphasia

(Head—"Syntactic Aphasia"; Goldstein—"Sensory Aphasia"; Luria—"Acoustic Aphasia"; Weisenburg and McBride—"Receptive Aphasia.")

This syndrome, the most common of the "fluent" aphasias, usually depends on a lesion in the posterior portion of the first temporal gyrus of the left hemisphere. The critical features of this syndrome are impaired auditory comprehension and fluently articulated but paraphasic speech. The impairment of auditory comprehension is evident even at the one-word level. The patient may repeat the examiner's words uncomprehendingly, or with paraphasic distortions. At severe levels, auditory comprehension may be zero, while paraphasia is so pervasive as to produce mean-

## SUBTEST SUMMARY PROFILE

NAME: **J.M.**                    DATE OF EXAM: **12-9-68**

| Category | Subtest | 0 | 10 | 20 | 30 | 40 | 50 | 60 | 70 | 80 | 90 | 100 |
|---|---|---|---|---|---|---|---|---|---|---|---|---|
| SEVERITY RATING | | | 0 | (✳) | | | | 2 | | 3 | 4 | 5 |
| FLUENCY | ARTICULATION RATING | | 1 | 2 | ✳ | 5 | 6 | | 7 | | | |
| | PHRASE LENGTH | | | ✳ | 3 | 4 | 5 | 6 | 7 | | | |
| | MELODIC LINE | | | 2 | 4 | | | 6 | 7 | | | |
| | VERBAL AGILITY | | 0 | 2 | 5 | ✳ | 8 | 9 | 11 | 13 | 14 | |
| AUDITORY COMPREHENSION | WORD DISCRIMINATION | 0 | 15 | 25 | 37 | 46 | 53 | 60 | 64 ✳ 67 | | 70 | 72 |
| | BODY-PART IDENTIFICATION | 0 | 1 | 5 | 10 | 13 | 15 | 16 | 17 | 18 | ✳ | 20 |
| | COMMANDS | 0 | 3 | 4 | 6 | 8 | 10 | 11 | 13 | 14 ✳ | | |
| | COMPLEX IDEATIONAL MATERIAL | | 0 | 2 | 3 | 4 | 5 | 6 | 8 | 9 ✳ | | 12 |
| NAMING | RESPONSIVE NAMING | | | 0 | 1 | 5 | 10 | 15 | 20 ✳ | | 27 | 30 |
| | CONFRONTATION NAMING | | 0 | 9 | 28 | 43 ✳ | | | 72 | 84 | 94 | 105   114 |
| | ANIMAL NAMING | | | | 0 | 1 | 2 | 3 | 4 | 6 ✳ | | 23 |
| ORAL READING | WORD READING | | | 0 | 1 | 3 | 7 | 15 ✳ | 21 | 26 | 30 | |
| | ORAL SENTENCE READING | | | | | 0 | 1 | ✳ | 4 | 7 | 9 | 10 |
| REPETITION | REPETITION OF WORDS | | 0 | 2 | 5 | ✳ | 8 | | 9 | | 10 | |
| | HIGH-PROBABILITY | | | 0 | 1 | | ✳ | 4 | 5 | 7 | 8 | |
| | LOW-PROBABILITY | | | | | ✳ | 1 | | 2 | 4 | 6 | 8 |
| PARAPHASIA | NEOLOGISTIC | 40 | 16 | 9 | 4 | 2 | 1 | ✳ | | | | |
| | LITERAL | 47 | 17 | 12 | 9 | 6 | 5 | 3 | 2 | 1 | ✳ | |
| | VERBAL | 40 | 23 | 18 | 15 | 12 | 9 | 7 | 4 | ✳ | 1 | 0 |
| | EXTENDED | 75 | 12 | 5 | 3 | 1 | ✳ | | | | | |
| AUTOMATIC SPEECH | AUTOMATIZED SEQUENCES | | 0 | 1 | 2 | 3 | ✳ | 6 | 7 | | 8 | |
| | RECITING | | | | 0 | ✳ | | | | 2 | | |
| READING COMPREHENSION | SYMBOL DISCRIMINATION | 0 | 2 | 5 | 7 | 8 | 9 | | ✳ | | | |
| | WORD RECOGNITION | 0 | 1 | 3 | 4 | 5 | 6 | ✳ | | 8 | | |
| | COMPREHENSION OF ORAL SPELLING | | | | 0 | 1 | | ✳ 3 | 4 | 6 | 7 | 8 |
| | WORD-PICTURE MATCHING | | | 0 | 1 | 4 | 6 | 8 | 9 ✳ | | | |
| | READING SENTENCES AND PARAGRAPHS | | | 0 | 1 | 2 | 3 | 4 | 5 | 6 | 7 ✳ | 10 |
| WRITING | MECHANICS | 1 | | 2 | | ✳ | | 4 | | 5 | | |
| | SERIAL WRITING | | 0 | 7 | 18 | 25 ✳ | 30 | 33 | 40 | 43 | 46 | 47 |
| | PRIMER-LEVEL DICTATION | | 0 | 1 | ✳ 4 | 6 | 9 | 11 | 13 | 14 | 15 | |
| | SPELLING TO DICTATION | | | | | ✳ | 1 | 2 | 3 | 5 | 7 | 10 |
| | WRITTEN CONFRONTATION NAMING | | | | 0 | 1 | 2 ✳ | | 6 | 7 | 9 | 10 |
| | SENTENCES TO DICTATION | | | | | | ✳ | 1 | 3 | 6 | 8 | 12 |
| | NARRATIVE WRITING | | ✳ | 1 | | | 2 | | | 3 | 4 | 5 |
| MUSIC | SINGING | | 0 | ✳ | | 2 | | | | | | |
| | RHYTHM | | 0 | ✳ | | | | 2 | | | | |
| SPATIAL AND COMPUTATIONAL | DRAWING TO COMMAND | 0 | 6 | 7 | 8 | 9 | 10 | 11 | 12 | | ✳ | |
| | STICK MEMORY | 0 | 3 | 4 | 6 | 7 | 8 | 9 | 10 | 11 | ✳ | 14 |
| | 3-D BLOCKS | 0 | | 2 | 4 | 5 | 6 | 7 | 8 | ✳ | 10 | |
| | TOTAL FINGERS | 0 | 54 | 70 | 81 | 93 | 100 | 108 | 120 | 130 | 141 ✳ | ✳ |
| | RIGHT-LEFT | 0 | 1 | 3 | 4 | 6 | 8 | 9 | 11 | ✳ | 16 | |
| | MAP ORIENTATION (OMITTED) | 0 | 2 | 5 | 6 | 9 | 11 | 13 | ✳ | 14 | | |
| | ARITHMETIC | | 0 | 2 | 4 | 8 | 11 | 14 ✳ | 17 | 21 | 27 | 32 |
| | CLOCK SETTING | 0 | 3 | 4 | 6 | | 8 | 9 | ✳ | 12 | | |
| | | 0 | 10 | 20 | 30 | 40 | 50 | 60 | 70 | 80 | 90 | 100 |

**Fig. 9.** Subtest score profile of a patient with Broca's aphasia.

### APHASIA SEVERITY RATING SCALE

0.  No usable speech or auditory comprehension.

1.  All communication is through fragmentary expression; great need for inference, questioning, and guessing by the listener. The range of information that can be exchanged is limited, and the listener carries the burden of communication.

2.  Conversation about familiar subjects is possible with help from the listener. There are frequent failures to convey the idea, but patient shares the burden of communication with the examiner.

3.  The patient can discuss <u>almost all everyday problems</u> with little or no assistance. Reduction of speech and/or comprehension, however, makes conversation about certain material difficult or impossible.

4.  Some obvious loss of fluency in speech or facility of comprehension, without significant limitation on ideas expressed or form of expression.

5.  Minimal discernible speech handicaps; patient may have subjective difficulties that are not apparent to listener.

### RATING SCALE PROFILE OF SPEECH CHARACTERISTICS

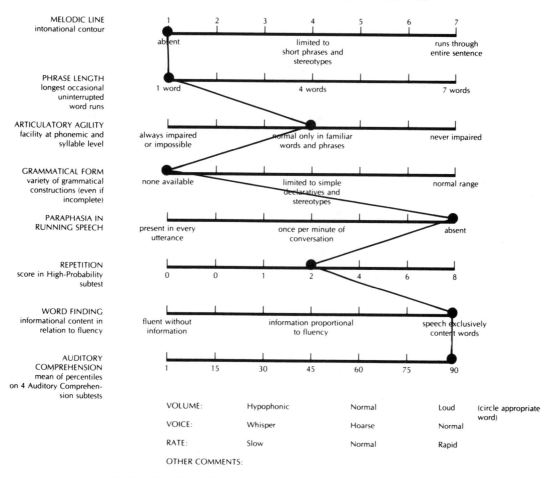

**Fig. 10.** Speech Profile ratings of a patient with Broca's aphasia.

ingless jargon. Paraphasia may include both sound transpositions (literal paraphasia) and word substitutions (verbal paraphasia). In addition, word-finding difficulty is an almost constant feature of this disorder, while reading and writing are usually severely impaired as well.

Though the grammar of these patients is often incorrect, there is usually free use of complex verb tenses, embedded subordinate clauses, and other departures from simple declarative word order. Their syntax therefore is described as "paragrammatic" rather than "agrammatic."

Repetition usually results in paraphasic distortion of the examiner's words, with the appearance of neologisms and irrelevant insertions. These patients often add a word or phrase or use a more complex form than that given—a feature termed "augmentation." Another frequent concomitant of this disorder is a press of speech, often at a rate greater than normal, while the patient is unaware of anything wrong with his speech.

A patient with Wernicke's aphasia may sound like a normal speaker from a distance, because of his fluency and the normal melodic contour of his speech. At milder levels, auditory comprehension difficulty is improved to the point at which only complex statements are misunderstood. Paraphasia, too, may become only an occasional feature, and the patient starts to demonstrate awareness of his own errors, by self correction and inhibition. Because the posterior location of the lesion usually spares the motor area, these patients may continue to use the right hand for writing and, in many cases, they preserve their natural handwriting, although the content of their written production is unintelligible. Occasional Wernicke's aphasics produce fluent, but paraphasic writing that parallels their speech in its disorganized, rambling style, in which there is repetitious use of certain words or phrases and a dearth of substantives and concrete action words. The following is a sample of writing obtained from such a patient:

> "His wife saw the wonting to wofin to a house with the umblelor. Then he left the wonding then he too to the womin and to the umbella up stairs. His wife carry it upstairs. Then the house did not go faster thern and tell go in the without within pain where it is whire in the herce in stock."

The theoretic model proposed for this defect is that Wernicke's area is the crossroad for all meaningful associations to sound patterns and for performances (such as reading and writing) that have been learned in conjunction with the auditory component of words. Its location, adjacent to the primary cortical auditory center (Heschl's gyrus), suggests that it plays the role of association area for audition, analogously with the other association areas, visual and motor, that are contiguous to the primary cortical end-stations for those modalities.

It is readily understandable that injury to such a center may reduce performances that depend on past and current auditory experience; however, one can only conjecture on the mechanism by which such injury may also produce paraphasia, excessively rapid speech, and anomia, while leaving syntactic automatisms relatively intact. Wernicke and others have suggested that paraphasia is the result of defective auditory monitoring of the speech output. This explanation fits well with the patient's unawareness of errors, but does not explain where the inappropriate speech comes from in the first place. Pressure of speech and resistance to interruption sometimes strike the listener as a result of the patient's failure to experience the "closure" that comes with the awareness of having finished expressing an idea. Depending on the patient's temperament and drive to express himself, he may press on blindly in speech, reaching for the elusive sense of having said what he intended.

CONFIGURATION OF TEST SCORES. The degree of severity of the Wernicke aphasic may fall at any level from "0" (no communication possible in either direction) to "4." A rating of "4" would be applied to a patient who, after extended, virtually normal conversation, breaks into occasional paraphasic irrelevancies. Like mild Broca's aphasics, such patients cannot be distinguished reliably from mild anomics at severity levels "4" and "5," where diagnostic distinctions tend to break down.

Figure 11 shows, in its shaded area, the range of ratings consistent with Wernicke's aphasia.

The Aphasia Subtest Summary Profile shows auditory comprehension and severity scores lower than fluency. Naming is also usu-

## RATING SCALE PROFILE OF SPEECH CHARACTERISTICS

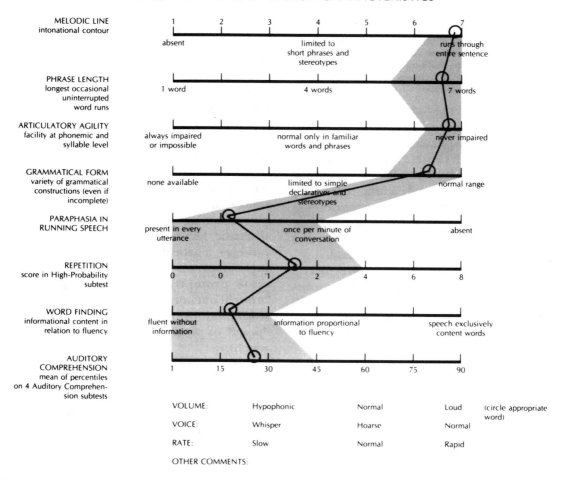

**Fig. 11.** Wernicke's aphasia. Shaded area indicates range of profile ratings compatible with this disorder. Heavy line indicates the mean of 14 representative cases.

ally below the fluency level. All of the paraphasia indicators are elevated. Repetition is commensurate with severity, and both reading and writing clusters are depressed.

A CASE OF WERNICKE'S APHASIA. A.M., a 56-year-old physician, suffered a vascular accident diagnosed as a thrombosis in the distribution of the left middle cerebral artery, with effects extending posteriorly to the angular gyrus. The episode occurred in January, 1963, 8 months prior to his examination. By the time he was seen, his initial right hemiparesis had cleared, leaving only a mild hyperreflexia on the right, along with a right homonymous hemianopia. Sensation was normal. On examination by Dr. Geschwind, A.M. was noted to present the classic picture of Wernicke's aphasia, with difficulty in all language

input and output modalities, but with fluent, easily articulated paraphasic speech.

The following transcript of the "cookie theft" narrative reveals the typical pattern of compound and complex sentence structures, which get nowhere because semantically meaningless sequences are juxtaposed. Paraphasia consists of totally irrelevant English words, neologisms, and repetitious overuse of phrases built around the words, "time" and "work."

> "Well this is . . . mother is away here working her work out o' here to get her better, but when she's looking, the two boys looking in the other part. One their small tile into her time here. She's working another time because she's getting, too. So the two boys work together an one is sneakin' around here, making his . . . work an' his further funnas his time he had. He an' the other fellow

were running around the work here, while mother another time she was doing that without everything wrong here. It isn't right, because she's making a time here of work time here, letting mother getting all wet here about something. The kids aren't right here because they don't just say one here and one here—that's all right, although the fellow here is breakin' between the two of them, they're comin' around too."

Examination of the Subtest Summary Profile for A.M. (Figure 12) reveals a severity rating of "1" and aphasia subscores at or near the zero level in all clusters representing purposeful use of linguistic skills, e.g., auditory comprehension, naming, reading, repetition, and writing. Thus, he might be considered a global aphasic from these scores alone, if we did not also see a high rating in fluency and a large count of paraphasias in extended utterances, which mark him as a Wernicke's aphasic. It should be noted that the opportunity for A.M. to produce paraphasias during formal testing was much reduced because the speech production tests were all abridged in view of the irrelevancy of his replies.

The scores on the subtests of the spatial-quantitative battery are uniformly low, in accordance with the clinical observations leading to the inference of a Sylvian lesion extending posteriorly towards the angular gyrus.

This profile of speech characteristics (Figure 13) is a classic one for Wernicke's aphasia with the four upper-scale ratings at or near the normal end and the four lower scales reflecting ratings of maximum abnormality.

### Anomia

(Head—"Nominal Aphasia"; Wepman—"Semantic Aphasia"; Goldstein—"Amnesic Aphasia.")

The syndromes of Wernicke's aphasia and of anomia do not have a sharp boundary, although the classic forms of each of these "fluent" aphasias are unmistakably distinct. Not only are there cases at every point along the continuum of symptoms between these two syndromes, but some patients, who appear initially as full-blown Wernicke aphasics, evolve into typical anomics in the course of their recovery.

The major feature of anomic aphasia is the prominence of word-finding difficulty in the context of fluent, grammatically well-formed speech. It differs from Wernicke's aphasia in the absence of literal and verbal paraphasia, and in the relative intactness of auditory comprehension. The classic anomic aphasic speaks freely, but with a dramatic emptiness of substantive words in his speech. In free conversation, some anomic aphasics are extremely facile in producing circumlocutions for their missing words. These circumlocutions may sound bizarre because of their vagueness, e.g., for "I had an operation on my head," one may hear, "I had one of them up there," or, with more specific circumlocutory terms, "I had a thing done up where your hair is." Testing of object-naming to confrontation will produce dramatic failures in extreme cases. Often, however, a patient whose conversation is strikingly empty of content, names most objects quite promptly, and a naming deficit is brought out only by pressing for less common words and for names of parts of objects (e.g., "point" of pencil, "teeth" of comb, "band" of watch).

While auditory comprehension is relatively good, the patient sometimes fails to recognize or accept a proffered word that he has been unable to evoke himself. For example, shown a wallet, the patient may say, "That's a purse." When asked if "wallet" would not be a better term, he may reject it, say it makes no difference which word is used or say, evasively, "You can call it that if you like." A study by Goodglass, Gleason, and Hyde (1970) reveals that these patients have significantly poorer comprehension of isolated nouns and verbs, with respect to their overall comprehension level, than do other types of patients.

Reading and writing may vary over a wide range from patient to patient. Anomia is often based on a temporal-parietal injury, which may extend into the angular gyrus, which is most sensitive for disturbances of written language. In these cases, severe alexia and agraphia are part of the picture. Other patients, however, read at a functional level and write as they speak. Occasionally, a patient of this type will spell orally or write a word that he cannot produce, suggesting that the spelled version of the word is learned and stored in parallel with the auditory model, but independently of it. Close examination of these cases shows that these acts of spelling are spo-

## SUBTEST SUMMARY PROFILE

NAME: **A.M.**                     DATE OF EXAM: **9-3-63**

| | | 0 | 10 | 20 | 30 | 40 | 50 | 60 | 70 | 80 | 90 | 100 |
|---|---|---|---|---|---|---|---|---|---|---|---|---|
| | PERCENTILES: | 0 | 10 | 20 | 30 | 40 | 50 | 60 | 70 | 80 | 90 | 100 |
| SEVERITY RATING | | | 0 | (*) | | | | 2 | | 3 | 4 | 5 |
| FLUENCY | ARTICULATION RATING | | 1 | 2 | 4 | 5 | 6 | | * | | | |
| | PHRASE LENGTH | | | 1 | 3 | 4 | 5 | 6 | 7 | | | |
| | MELODIC LINE | | 1 | 2 | 4 | | 6 | 7 | | | | |
| | VERBAL AGILITY (OMITTED) | | 0 | 2 | 5 | 6 | 8 | 9 | 11 | 13 | 14 | |
| AUDITORY COMPREHENSION | WORD DISCRIMINATION | * | 15 | 25 | 37 | 46 | 53 | 60 | 64 | 67 | 70 | 72 |
| | BODY-PART IDENTIFICATION | | 1 | 5 | 10 | 13 | 15 | 16 | 17 | 18 | | 20 |
| | COMMANDS | 0 | 3 | 4 | 6 | 8 | 10 | 11 | 13 | 14 | 15 | |
| | COMPLEX IDEATIONAL MATERIAL | * | 2 | 3 | 4 | 5 | 6 | 8 | 9 | 11 | 12 | |
| NAMING | RESPONSIVE NAMING | | | | * | 1 | 5 | 10 | 15 | 20 | 24 | 27 | 30 |
| | CONFRONTATION NAMING | | 9 | 28 | 43 | 60 | 72 | 84 | 94 | 105 | 114 | |
| | ANIMAL NAMING | | | | * | 1 | 2 | 3 | 4 | 6 | 9 | 23 |
| ORAL READING | WORD READING | | | * | 1 | 3 | 7 | 15 | 21 | 26 | 30 | |
| | ORAL SENTENCE READING | | | | * | 1 | 2 | 4 | 7 | 9 | 10 | |
| REPETITION | REPETITION OF WORDS | 0 | * | 2 | 5 | 7 | 8 | | 9 | | 10 | |
| | HIGH-PROBABILITY | | | * | 1 | | 2 | 4 | 5 | 7 | 8 | |
| | LOW-PROBABILITY | | | | * | 1 | | 2 | 4 | 6 | 8 | |
| PARAPHASIA | NEOLOGISTIC | 40 | 16 | 9 | 4 | 2 | 1 | * | | | | |
| | LITERAL | 47 | 17 | 12 | 9 | 6 | 5 | 3 | 2 | 1 | * | |
| | VERBAL | 40 | 23 | 18 | 15 | 12 | 9 | 7 | 4 | 3 | * | 0 |
| | EXTENDED | 75 | 12 | * | 3 | 1 | 0 | | | | | |
| AUTOMATIC SPEECH | AUTOMATIZED SEQUENCES | | 0 | * | 2 | 3 | 4 | 6 | 7 | | 8 | |
| | RECITING | | | | * | 1 | | | | 2 | | |
| READING COMPREHENSION | SYMBOL DISCRIMINATION | 0 | 2 | 5 | 7 | 8 | 9 | | 10 | | | |
| | WORD RECOGNITION | * | 1 | 3 | 4 | 5 | 6 | 7 | | 8 | | |
| | COMPREHENSION OF ORAL SPELLING | | | | * | 1 | | 3 | 4 | 6 | 7 | 8 |
| | WORD-PICTURE MATCHING | | * | 1 | 4 | 6 | 8 | 9 | | 10 | | |
| | READING SENTENCES AND PARAGRAPHS | * | 1 | 2 | 3 | 4 | 5 | 6 | 7 | 8 | 10 | |
| WRITING | MECHANICS | * | | 2 | | 3 | | 4 | | 5 | | |
| | SERIAL WRITING | | 0 | 7 | 18* | 25 | 30 | 33 | 40 | 43 | 46 | 47 |
| | PRIMER-LEVEL DICTATION | | * | 1 | 4 | 6 | 9 | 11 | 13 | 14 | 15 | |
| | SPELLING TO DICTATION | | | | | * | 1 | 2 | 3 | 5 | 7 | 10 |
| | WRITTEN CONFRONTATION NAMING | | | | * | 1 | 2 | 3 | 6 | 7 | 9 | 10 |
| | SENTENCES TO DICTATION | | | | | * | 1 | 3 | 6 | 8 | 12 | |
| | NARRATIVE WRITING | | 0 | * | | | 2 | | | 3 | 4 | 5 |
| MUSIC | SINGING | | 0 | 1 | | * | | | | | | |
| | RHYTHM | | 0 | 1 | | | | | * | | | |
| SPATIAL AND COMPUTATIONAL | DRAWING TO COMMAND | * | 6 | 7 | 8 | 9 | 10 | 11 | 12 | | 13 | |
| | STICK MEMORY | 0 | * | 4 | 6 | 7 | 8 | 9 | 10 | 11 | 13 | 14 |
| | 3-D BLOCKS | | 0 | 2 | 4 | 5 | 6 | 7 | 8 | 9 | 10 | |
| | TOTAL FINGERS | 0 | 54 | 70 | 81 | 93 | 100 | 108 | 120 | 130 | 141 | 152 |
| | RIGHT-LEFT | 0 | 1 | 3 | 4 | 6 | * | 9 | 11 | 14 | 16 | |
| | MAP ORIENTATION (OMITTED) | 0 | 2 | 5 | 6 | 9 | 11 | 13 | | 14 | | |
| | ARITHMETIC | | * | 2 | 4 | 8 | 11 | 14 | 17 | 21 | 27 | 32 |
| | CLOCK SETTING | 0 | * | 4 | 6 | | 8 | 9 | 10 | 12 | | |
| | | 0 | 10 | 20 | 30 | 40 | 50 | 60 | 70 | 80 | 90 | 100 |

**Fig. 12.** Subtest score profile of a patient with Wernicke's aphasia.

## APHASIA SEVERITY RATING SCALE

0. No usable speech or auditory comprehension.

1. All communication is through fragmentary expression; great need for inference, questioning, and guessing by the listener. The range of information that can be exchanged is limited, and the listener carries the burden of communication.

2. Conversation about familiar subjects is possible with help from the listener. There are frequent failures to convey the idea, but patient shares the burden of communication with the examiner.

3. The patient can discuss <u>almost all everyday problems</u> with little or no assistance. Reduction of speech and/or comprehension, however, makes conversation about certain material difficult or impossible.

4. Some obvious loss of fluency in speech or facility of comprehension, without significant limitation on ideas expressed or form of expression.

5. Minimal discernible speech handicaps; patient may have subjective difficulties that are not apparent to listener.

### RATING SCALE PROFILE OF SPEECH CHARACTERISTICS

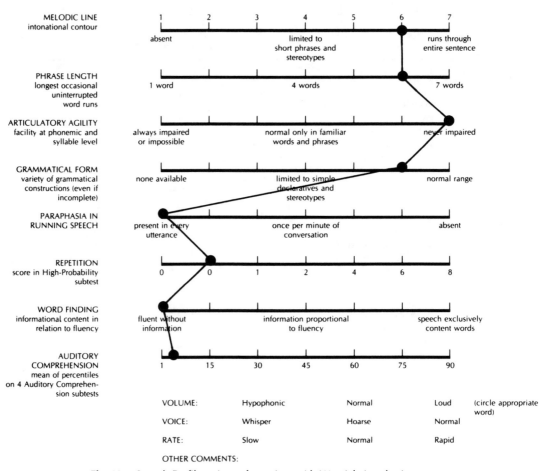

**Fig. 13.** Speech Profile ratings of a patient with Wernicke's aphasia.

radic and that their writing of object-names is not much better than their verbalization. In spite of its frequent association with angular gyrus lesions, anomia is the least reliably localizable of the aphasic syndromes. It is commonly the first language disturbance with growing brain tumors that may exert pressure, though remote from the recognized language areas.

CONFIGURATION OF TEST SCORES. Anomic aphasics of severe degree are quite rare, and the severity rating of a patient of this type is usually "3" or "4." The speech profile of the classic form of this disorder is distinguished from a normal profile only by the word-finding scale, which is displaced towards the extreme of "fluent without information." The range of ratings consistent with anomic aphasia is included in the shaded area of Figure 14.

The Aphasia Subtest Summary Profile shows high fluency and auditory comprehension scores as well as a severity rating above the midpoint of the scales. Visual Confrontation Naming is usually lower than the foregoing scores, but only in extreme cases does it fall below the fiftieth percentile. Paraphasia scores are low, except for "other" or "extended" paraphasia (last column), which may reflect occurrences of circumlocution during the test. Repetition is high, while reading and writing scores are unpredictable.

A CASE OF ANOMIC APHASIA. R.D. was a 54-year-old, right-handed man who, though he had only 8 years of formal schooling, had worked as a ship designer and had written a

## RATING SCALE PROFILE OF SPEECH CHARACTERISTICS

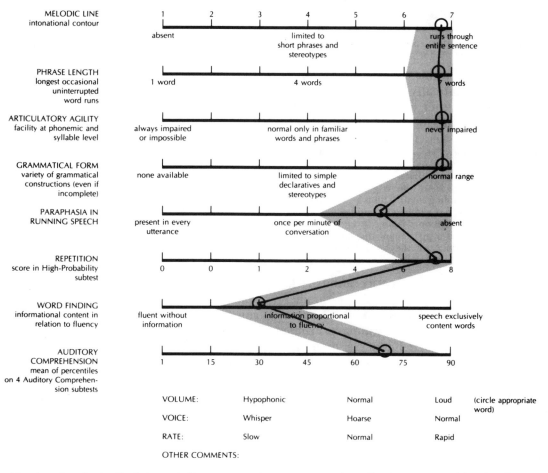

**Fig. 14.** Anomic aphasia. Shaded area indicates range of ratings on Speech Profile characteristic of this disorder. Heavy line represents mean ratings of ten representative anomic aphasics.

small book on ship design. He had suffered the onset of a right hemiplegia and speech difficulty without unconsciousness 3 months prior to his admission to the aphasia unit. By the time of his admission, his motor status had improved, with only residual weakness of his right arm. There was cortical sensory loss in the right arm only. An arteriogram revealed a complete occlusion of the left middle cerebral artery, but a radioactive brain scan revealed a lesion confined to the left parieto-occipital region.

The neurologist's examination found his spontaneous speech clear, fluent, and in full sentences, but reduced in rate and showing obvious word-finding difficulty. He was described as severely alexic and agraphic, having right-left confusion and apraxia for facial movements.

An example of his capacity for sentence organization from his free conversation is the following response to a question about the onset of his illness. "For three days, it was just a little bit here, then, all of a sudden, it just spread all over."

The sentences in his "cookie theft" narrative are grammatically somewhat simpler, being strung together by "and" connections. This narrative shows most strikingly the word-finding difficulty and the substitution of indefinites for nouns that he cannot evoke.

> "This is a boy and that's a boy an' that's a . . . thing! (Laughs.) An' this is goin' off pretty soon (points to toppling stool). This is a . . . a place that this is mostly in (Examiner: "Could you name the room . . . a bathroom?") No . . . kitchen . . . kitchen. An' this is a girl . . . an' that something that they're running an' they've got the water going down here . . ."

The patient received a severity rating of "2," indicating that conversation about familiar subjects is possible with help from the listener. Inspection of the Subtest Summary Profile (Figure 15) reveals that fluency is high and word finding is low, a configuration consistent with any of the posterior aphasias. Looking at the auditory comprehension scales, we note that, in spite of failure in word discrimination and body-part comprehension, these two scores lie slightly above the patient's general severity level, while the more complex comprehension scales are at near-normal levels. The severity of the aphasia seems chiefly due

to the depressed naming scores, which (except for responsive naming) fall *lower* on the percentile scale than does the severity rating and certainly well below the comprehension rating. This makes anomic aphasia the best-fitting syndrome. Conduction aphasia is excluded by the high repetition cluster and the absence of literal paraphasias.

The Subtest Summary Profile also reflects the severe impairment of written language noted by the neurologist. Both reading and writing clusters lie entirely below the oral language scores. This configuration is not a constant feature in anomic aphasia. It indicates a lesion implicating the posterior temporoparietal region (angular gyrus), which is also reflected in poor finger localization, right-left confusion, and acalculia on the spatial and quantitative tests.

Inspection of the Rating Scale Profile of Speech Characteristics (Figure 16) shows some deviation from the classic profile of anomia, in that some minimal articulatory deficit and restriction in variety of grammatical form are noted. Verbal paraphasias occur somewhat more in this patient's speech than in classic forms of anomia, but the word-finding difficulty itself is clearly indicated.

### Conduction Aphasia

(Goldstein—"Central Aphasia"; Luria—"Afferent Motor Aphasia.")

This is the name applied to the syndrome in which repetition is disproportionately severely impaired in relation to the level of fluency in spontaneous speech and to the near normal level of auditory comprehension. While it is considered one of the "fluent" aphasias, the fluency may be restricted to brief runs of speech. In these cases, the patients are unlike Broca's aphasics in that they usually produce well-articulated sequences of English phonemes with normal intonation and initiate a variety of syntactic patterns. The outstanding speech difficulty is in the proper choice and sequencing of their phonemes, so that *literal paraphasia* repeatedly interferes with production. Sometimes the patient's struggle with his literal paraphasia results in an output like that of a Broca's aphasic, and it may be difficult to differentiate these two types of

**SUBTEST SUMMARY PROFILE**

NAME: **R.D.**   DATE OF EXAM: **7-20-66**

| | | 0 | 10 | 20 | 30 | 40 | 50 | 60 | 70 | 80 | 90 | 100 |
|---|---|---|---|---|---|---|---|---|---|---|---|---|
| | PERCENTILES: | | | | | | | | | | | |
| SEVERITY RATING | | | 0 | 1 | | | | (✶) | | 3 | 4 | 5 |
| FLUENCY | ARTICULATION RATING | | 1 | 2 | 4 | 5 | 6 | | 7 | | | |
| | PHRASE LENGTH | | | 1 | 3 | 4 | 5 | 6 | | | | |
| | MELODIC LINE | | 1 | 2 | 4 | | 6 | | | | | |
| | VERBAL AGILITY | | 0 | 2 | 5 | 6 | 8 | 9 | 11 | | 14 | |
| AUDITORY COMPREHENSION | WORD DISCRIMINATION | 0 | 15 | 25 | 37 | 46 | | 60 | 64 | 67 | 70 | 72 |
| | BODY-PART IDENTIFICATION | 0 | 1 | 5 | 10 | 13 | | 16 | 17 | 18 | | 20 |
| | COMMANDS | 0 | 3 | 4 | 6 | 8 | 10 | 11 | 13 | | | |
| | COMPLEX IDEATIONAL MATERIAL | | 0 | 2 | 3 | 4 | 5 | 6 | 8 | 9 | 11 | 12 |
| NAMING | RESPONSIVE NAMING | | | 0 | 1 | 5 | 10 | 15 | 20 | | | 30 |
| | CONFRONTATION NAMING | | 0 | 9 | 28 | | | 60 | 72 | 84 | 94 | 105 | 114 |
| | ANIMAL NAMING | | | | 0 | 1 | 2 | 3 | | 6 | 9 | 23 |
| ORAL READING | WORD READING | | | | | 1 | 3 | 7 | 15 | 21 | 26 | 30 |
| | ORAL SENTENCE READING | | | | | | 1 | 2 | 4 | 7 | 9 | 10 |
| REPETITION | REPETITION OF WORDS | | 0 | 2 | 5 | 7 | 8 | | 9 | | | |
| | HIGH-PROBABILITY | | | 0 | 1 | | 2 | 4 | 5 | 7 | | |
| | LOW-PROBABILITY | | | | 0 | 1 | | | 2 | 4 | 6 | 8 |
| PARAPHASIA | NEOLOGISTIC | 40 | 16 | 9 | 4 | 2 | 1 | | | | | |
| | LITERAL | 47 | 17 | 12 | 9 | 6 | 5 | 3 | 2 | 1 | | |
| | VERBAL | 40 | 23 | 18 | 15 | 12 | 9 | 7 | 4 | 3 | 1 | 0 |
| | EXTENDED | 75 | 12 | 5 | | 1 | 0 | | | | | |
| AUTOMATIC SPEECH | AUTOMATIZED SEQUENCES | | 0 | 1 | 2 | 3 | 4 | | 7 | | 8 | |
| | RECITING | | | | 0 | 1 | | | | | | |
| READING COMPREHENSION | SYMBOL DISCRIMINATION | 0 | 2 | 5 | | 8 | 9 | | 10 | | | |
| | WORD RECOGNITION | 0 | 1 | | 4 | 5 | 6 | 7 | | 8 | | |
| | COMPREHENSION OF ORAL SPELLING | | | | | 1 | | 3 | 4 | 6 | 7 | 8 |
| | WORD-PICTURE MATCHING | | 0 | 1 | 4 | | 8 | 9 | | 10 | | |
| | READING SENTENCES AND PARAGRAPHS | | 1 | 2 | 3 | 4 | 5 | 6 | 7 | 8 | 10 |
| WRITING | MECHANICS | | | 2 | | 3 | | 4 | | 5 | | |
| | SERIAL WRITING | | 0 | 7 | 18 | 25 | 30 | 33 | 40 | 43 | 46 | 47 |
| | PRIMER-LEVEL DICTATION | | | 1 | 4 | 6 | 9 | 11 | 13 | 14 | 15 | |
| | SPELLING TO DICTATION | | | | | | 1 | 2 | 3 | 5 | 7 | 10 |
| | WRITTEN CONFRONTATION NAMING | | | | | 1 | 2 | 3 | 6 | 7 | 9 | 10 |
| | SENTENCES TO DICTATION | | | | | | | 1 | 3 | 6 | 8 | 12 |
| | NARRATIVE WRITING | | 1 | | | | 2 | | | 3 | 4 | 5 |
| MUSIC | SINGING | | 0 | | | 2 | | | | | | |
| | RHYTHM | | 0 | | | | | 2 | | | | |
| SPATIAL AND COMPUTATIONAL | DRAWING TO COMMAND | 0 | 6 | 7 | 8 | 9 | 10 | | 12 | | 13 | |
| | STICK MEMORY | 0 | 3 | | 6 | 7 | 8 | 9 | 10 | 11 | 13 | 14 |
| | 3-D BLOCKS | | 0 | 2 | 4 | 5 | 6 | 7 | | | 10 | |
| | TOTAL FINGERS | 0 | 54 | 70 | 81 | 93 | 100 | 108 | 120 | 130 | 141 | 152 |
| | RIGHT-LEFT | 0 | 1 | 3 | 4 | 6 | 8 | 9 | 11 | 14 | 16 | |
| | MAP ORIENTATION   (OMITTED) | 0 | 2 | 5 | 6 | 9 | 11 | 13 | | 14 | | |
| | ARITHMETIC | | | 2 | 4 | 8 | 11 | 14 | 17 | 21 | 27 | 32 |
| | CLOCK SETTING | 0 | 3 | 4 | 6 | | 8 | 9 | 10 | 12 | | |
| | | 0 | 10 | 20 | 30 | 40 | 50 | 60 | 70 | 80 | 90 | 100 |

**Fig. 15.** Subtest score profile of a patient with anomic aphasia.

## APHASIA SEVERITY RATING SCALE

0. No usable speech or auditory comprehension.

1. All communication is through fragmentary expression; great need for inference, questioning, and guessing by the listener. The range of information that can be exchanged is limited, and the listener carries the burden of communication.

2. Conversation about familiar subjects is possible with help from the listener. There are frequent failures to convey the idea, but patient shares the burden of communication with the examiner.

3. The patient can discuss <u>almost all everyday problems</u> with little or no assistance. Reduction of speech and/or comprehension, however, makes conversation about certain material difficult or impossible.

4. Some obvious loss of fluency in speech or facility of comprehension, without significant limitation on ideas expressed or form of expression.

5. Minimal discernible speech handicaps; patient may have subjective difficulties that are not apparent to listener.

## RATING SCALE PROFILE OF SPEECH CHARACTERISTICS

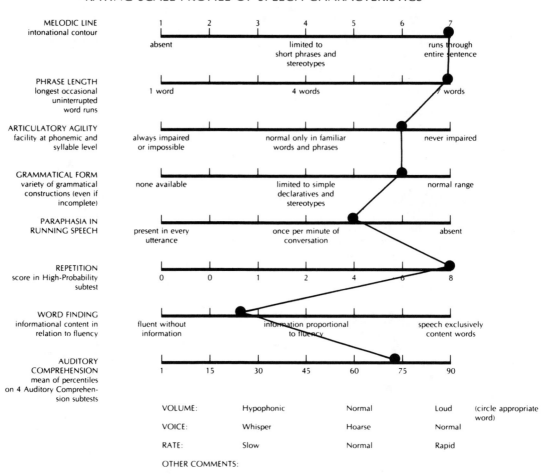

**Fig. 16.** Speech Profile ratings of a patient with anomic aphasia.

aphasia on the basis of the articulation rating scale. In the more fluent conduction aphasic, an *anomic* component is very prominent, and the patient may run along fluently until he encounters a substantive or a principal verb, at which point he struggles paraphasically, with repeated aproximations, to untangle the sounds of this word. This "zeroing in" behavior is referred to as "conduite d'approche" in the French literature. Unlike the Wernicke aphasic, the conduction aphasic is acutely aware of his inaccuracy and rejects his incorrect efforts.

It is primarily in repetition that we see literal paraphasic intrusions interfering with the intended output. While familiar single words and short, conversational expressions rarely present difficulty for repetition, the conduction aphasic is baffled by polysyllabic words, and has particular difficulty with sentences composed primarily of pronouns and grammatical functors, as illustrated in Chapter 5 under "Repetition Tests for Conduction Aphasia." Whereas the articulation of a Broca's aphasic is always aided by a model for repetition, the reverse is true for the conduction aphasic.

One of the striking phenomena in repetition difficulties is the difference between numbers and other speech forms. These patients often respond perfectly normally to the request for number repetition, in striking contrast to their groping attempts at other words. Moreover, errors with number repetition take the form of verbal paraphasia (word-substitution) rather than literal paraphasia. When numbers are combined with words (e.g., "84 divided by 7 equals 12"), the contrast between them may emerge dramatically. (See supplementary tests for repetition in Chapter 5).

The auditory comprehension of these patients may be completely intact. They were found to have a normal mean score in auditory comprehension vocabulary—superior to that of anomics.

Conduction aphasia is attributed by some (e.g., Geschwind, 1965) to a lesion in the arcuate fasciculus—a fiber pathway believed to carry information from Wernicke's area to Broca's area. It is affected by a lesion deep to the supramarginal gyrus, but lesions may also be found in the superior temporal gyrus or in the insula (Damasio and Damasio, 1980).

CONFIGURATION OF TEST SCORES. Conduction aphasics are not readily diagnosable at the most severe levels (0 to 1) since, if their speech is very sparse, they may resemble Broca's aphasics or, if they are more fluent, they may have some of the impaired comprehension and verbal and neologistic paraphasia of Wernicke aphasics. Unambiguous cases of this syndrome may range from severity level "2" to "4." Their profiles on the speech characteristics scale are variable at several points, notably for phrase length and articulation, but they show a distinct deficit on the repetition scales (Figure 17).

Paraphasia in running speech may occur in some patients who do not bother to self correct. Others will always stop at an error, interrupting their flow. The auditory comprehension scale ranges from moderate impairment to normal.

On the Subtest Summary Profile of the Diagnostic Aphasia Test, auditory comprehension is on a par with or superior to severity and fluency levels. Repetition is depressed, especially at the sentence level. The paraphasia cluster shows an elevation in literal paraphasia and sometimes in neologistic paraphasia. Reading comprehension and writing scores are usually commensurate with the severity rating.

A CASE OF CONDUCTION APHASIA. K.L. was a 20-year-old male, high school graduate who, while at a U.S. Air Force base, suffered a 22-caliber bullet wound in the head on January 16, 1964, 2 months prior to this examination. The bullet entered the left lower midparietal region and crossed the midline, coming to rest in the right parietal lobe. There were bilateral intracerebral hematomas and bone fragments in the path of the bullet. Bilateral craniotomy was performed to remove the bullet, drain and debride the wound.

When seen 2 months later, he had a very mild right-sided weakness, diminished position sense, and increased two-point discrimination threshold in both hands with astereognosis bilaterally. His speech was described as fluent with good rhythm and occasional long sentences in free conversation. In repetition, however, he appeared dysarthric and spoke

### RATING SCALE PROFILE OF SPEECH CHARACTERISTICS

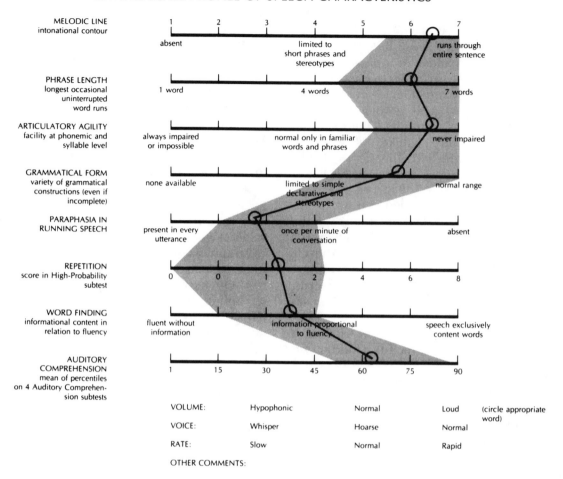

**Fig. 17.** Conduction aphasia. Shaded area indicates range of Speech Profile ratings compatible with this disorder. Heavy line represents mean ratings for ten representative patients.

with effort. He was considered a conduction aphasic. His gunshot wound also was located precisely in a position to interfere with the path of the arcuate fasciculus, consistent with the anatomic rationale for conduction aphasia.

The following transcript of narrative description of the "cookie theft" picture is typical of his speech. It illustrates his capacity for extended grammatical runs of speech, his generally self-corrected word-finding slips, and the phonemic substitutions that appear, principally in substantives, in a general context of facile articulation.

"Well this um . . . somebody's . . . ah mahther is takin the . . . washin' the dayshes an' the water . . . the water is falling . . . is flowing all over the place, an' the kids sneaking' out in back behind her, takin' the cookies in the . . . out of the top in the . . . what do you call that? (Examiner: "Shelf?")

Yes . . . and there's a . . . then the girl . . . not the girl . . . the boy who's getting the cookies is on this ah . . . strool an' startin' to fall off. That's about all I see."

Inspection of the Rating Scale Profile of Speech Characteristics (Figure 18) reveals ratings at or near the normal position on all scales except those for paraphasia and word finding. His atypically high performance on High-Probability Sentence Repetition puts him above the range, observed in the performance of 10 prototypical conduction aphasics (Figure 17). His severity rating was "3." This, in conjunction with the normal auditory comprehension score, is typical for conduction aphasia. The Subtest Summary Profile (Figure 19) shows that, while absolute scores for repetition are only moderately depressed, they are lower than the fluency and auditory comprehension levels. Moreover, the count of literal paraphasias is by far the highest in the paraphasia group. This patient performs at the top of our reading scale, but earns only a score of "1" in spelling from dictation. Nevertheless, he could write an incomplete but relevant sentence about the cookie theft in which, through his poor spelling, omissions, and partly illegible letters, a well-formulated sentence could be discerned.

The patient's scores on the spatial-quantitative subtests are all within the normal range.

## Transcortical Sensory Aphasia

This syndrome, which is rather rare, is characterized by the remarkable preservation of repetition in the context of the features of a severe Wernicke's aphasia. The postulated pathophysiology of this syndrome (Geschwind, Segarra, and Quadfasel, 1968) is that the auditory-vocal mechanism of the speech area, represented by the Wernicke-Broca area complex, is spared, but cut off posteriorly from the rest of the brain by a band of infarcted brain tissue. Lesions of this type (referred to as "watershed" lesions) may be produced by vascular insufficiency. The rationale for the set of symptoms is that Wernicke's area can perform its operations of auditory analysis and classification and pass its information along to an intact Broca's area to permit repetition. The isolation of this portion of the speech system, however, prevents any interaction between the knowledge, intention, and perceptions of the rest of the brain and those of the isolated speech mechanism.

The typical patient with this disorder converses with well-articulated, but irrelevant paraphasia that may include both actual English words and neologisms. He is usually unable to name to confrontation and may offer grossly irrelevant responses when so stimulated. These patients often echo the examiner's words instead of replying. Their ability to repeat is not limited to echoing, however, as they may, on request, listen to and repeat back correctly sentences of considerable length and complexity.

Along with the remarkable sparing of repetition, there is an unusual preservation of memorized material. Patients of this group may recite perfectly the Lord's Prayer or other familiar passages. They also sing, with the words, any songs that were known to them premorbidly, once given a start.

Written language is severely impaired both for reading and writing.

APPEARANCE OF TEST PROFILE. The severity rating of patients with transcortical sensory aphasia is most likely to be at level "1" or "2." The appearance of their Rating Scale Profile of Speech Characteristics does not differ from that of Wernicke's aphasia, except for their intact repetition. The Subtest Summary Profile, however, will show all repetition scores elevated with respect to severity and auditory comprehension, with the remainder of the profile similar to that of Wernicke's aphasia.

A CASE OF TRANSCORTICAL SENSORY APHASIA. C.N. was a 49-year-old male whose educational and occupational backgrounds were unknown. He had been injured in an automobile accident in August, 1963, 16 months prior to his examination at the Boston VA Hospital. He had suffered a left temporoparietal hematoma, which had been removed, and he had a plate over his skull defect. He had a severe hemiplegia.

On examination, he was socially appropriate and aware of his difficulty. His speech was described as normal in rate, rhythm, and length of phrases, but with an emptiness of relevant substantives, and runs of irrelevant jargon of English and neologistic words. He trailed off without completing the sense of his sentences. Auditory comprehension was moderately impaired, but would deteriorate during the course of a testing session. He was severely alexic and agraphic and completely apraxic. The words "right" and "left" were devoid of meaning to him, although he could find his way easily about the hospital.

The striking feature of this patient was his remarkable ability to repeat long sentences, even foreign phrases, correctly in the face of his profound naming difficulty and paraphasia in other than repetition responses. He also had a strong urge to echo, which could be restrained only with repeated instructions.

Some examples of his confabulatory responses to naming of visual stimuli are:

## APHASIA SEVERITY RATING SCALE

0. No usable speech or auditory comprehension.

1. All communication is through fragmentary expression; great need for inference, questioning, and guessing by the listener. The range of information that can be exchanged is limited, and the listener carries the burden of communication.

2. Conversation about familiar subjects is possible with help from the listener. There are frequent failures to convey the idea, but patient shares the burden of communication with the examiner.

3. The patient can discuss almost all everyday problems with little or no assistance. Reduction of speech and/or comprehension, however, makes conversation about certain material difficult or impossible.

4. Some obvious loss of fluency in speech or facility of comprehension, without significant limitation on ideas expressed or form of expression.

5. Minimal discernible speech handicaps; patient may have subjective difficulties that are not apparent to listener.

## RATING SCALE PROFILE OF SPEECH CHARACTERISTICS

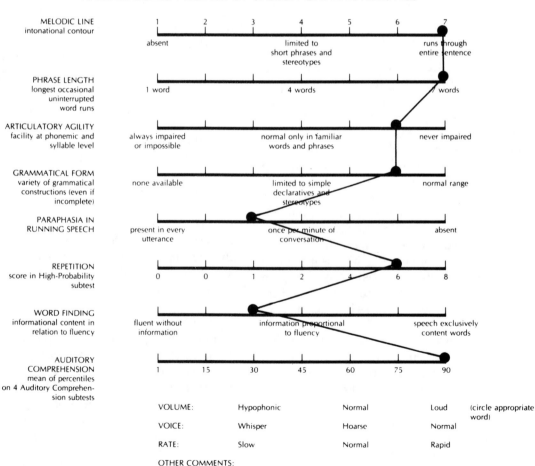

**Fig. 18.** Speech Profile ratings of a patient with conduction aphasia.

## SUBTEST SUMMARY PROFILE

NAME: **K.L.**   DATE OF EXAM: **3-26-64**

| | Subtest | 0 | 10 | 20 | 30 | 40 | 50 | 60 | 70 | 80 | 90 | 100 |
|---|---|---|---|---|---|---|---|---|---|---|---|---|
| **SEVERITY RATING** | | | 0 | 1 | | | | 2 | | (3) | 4 | 5 |
| **FLUENCY** | ARTICULATION RATING | | 1 | 2 | 4 | 5 | 6 | | | | | |
| | PHRASE LENGTH | | | 1 | 3 | 4 | 5 | 6 | | | | |
| | MELODIC LINE | | 1 | 2 | 4 | | 6 | | | | | |
| | VERBAL AGILITY | | 0 | 2 | 5 | 6 | | 9 | 11 | 13 | 14 | |
| **AUDITORY COMPREHENSION** | WORD DISCRIMINATION | 0 | 15 | 25 | 37 | 46 | 53 | 60 | 64 | 67 | 70 | 72 |
| | BODY-PART IDENTIFICATION | 0 | 1 | 5 | 10 | 13 | 15 | 16 | 17 | 18 | | 20 |
| | COMMANDS | 0 | 3 | 4 | 6 | 8 | 10 | 11 | 13 | 14 | | |
| | COMPLEX IDEATIONAL MATERIAL | | 0 | 2 | 3 | 4 | 5 | 6 | 8 | 9 | | 12 |
| **NAMING** | RESPONSIVE NAMING | | | 0 | 1 | 5 | 10 | 15 | 20 | 24 | 27 | 30 |
| | CONFRONTATION NAMING | | 0 | 9 | 28 | 43 | 60 | 72 | 84 | 94 | 105 | 114 |
| | ANIMAL NAMING | | | 0 | 1 | 2 | 3 | 4 | 6 | | | 23 |
| **ORAL READING** | WORD READING | | | 0 | 1 | 3 | 7 | 15 | 21 | 26 | 30 | |
| | ORAL SENTENCE READING | | | | 0 | 1 | 2 | 4 | 7 | | 9 | 10 |
| **REPETITION** | REPETITION OF WORDS | | 0 | 2 | 5 | 7 | | | 9 | | 10 | |
| | HIGH-PROBABILITY | | | 0 | 1 | | 2 | 4 | 5 | 7 | 8 | |
| | LOW-PROBABILITY | | | | 0 | 1 | | | 2 | 4 | 6 | 8 |
| **PARAPHASIA** | NEOLOGISTIC | 40 | 16 | 9 | 4 | 2 | 1 | | 0 | | | |
| | LITERAL | 47 | 17 | 12 | 9 | 6 | 5 | 3 | 2 | 1 | 0 | |
| | VERBAL | 40 | 23 | 18 | 15 | 12 | 9 | 7 | 4 | 3 | 1 | 0 |
| | EXTENDED | 75 | 12 | 5 | 3 | 1 | | | | | | |
| **AUTOMATIC SPEECH** | AUTOMATIZED SEQUENCES | | 0 | 1 | 2 | 3 | 4 | 6 | | | 8 | |
| | RECITING | | | | 0 | | | | | 2 | | |
| **READING COMPREHENSION** | SYMBOL DISCRIMINATION | 0 | 2 | 5 | 7 | 8 | 9 | | | | | |
| | WORD RECOGNITION | 0 | 1 | 3 | 4 | 5 | 6 | 7 | | | | |
| | COMPREHENSION OF ORAL SPELLING | | | | 0 | 1 | | 3 | 4 | 6 | 7 | |
| | WORD-PICTURE MATCHING | | | 0 | 1 | 4 | 6 | 8 | 9 | | | |
| | READING SENTENCES AND PARAGRAPHS | | | 0 | 1 | 2 | 3 | 4 | 5 | 6 | 7 | 8 / 10 |
| **WRITING** | MECHANICS | 1 | | | | 3 | | 4 | | 5 | | |
| | SERIAL WRITING | | 0 | 7 | 18 | 25 | 30 | 33 | 40 | 43 | 46 | 47 |
| | PRIMER-LEVEL DICTATION | | 0 | 1 | 4 | 6 | 9 | 11 | 13 | 14 | | |
| | SPELLING TO DICTATION | | | | | 0 | | 2 | 3 | 5 | 7 | 10 |
| | WRITTEN CONFRONTATION NAMING | | | 0 | 1 | 2 | 3 | | | 7 | 9 | 10 |
| | SENTENCES TO DICTATION | | | | | | 0 | 1 | | 6 | 8 | 12 |
| | NARRATIVE WRITING | | 0 | 1 | | | | | | 3 | 4 | 5 |
| **MUSIC** | SINGING | | 0 | | | 2 | | | | | | |
| | RHYTHM | | 0 | 1 | | | | | | | | |
| **SPATIAL AND COMPUTATIONAL** | DRAWING TO COMMAND | 0 | 6 | 7 | 8 | 9 | 10 | 11 | 12 | | 13 | |
| | STICK MEMORY | 0 | 3 | 4 | 6 | 7 | 8 | 9 | 10 | 11 | 13 | 14 |
| | 3-D BLOCKS | | 0 | 2 | 4 | 5 | 6 | 7 | 8 | 9 | 10 | |
| | TOTAL FINGERS | 0 | 54 | 70 | 81 | 93 | 100 | 108 | 120 | 130 | 141 | 152 |
| | RIGHT-LEFT | 0 | 1 | 3 | 4 | 6 | 8 | 9 | 11 | 14 | 16 | |
| | MAP ORIENTATION | 0 | 2 | 5 | 6 | 9 | 11 | 13 | | 14 | | |
| | ARITHMETIC | | 0 | 2 | 4 | 8 | 11 | 14 | 17 | 21 | 27 | 32 |
| | CLOCK SETTING | 0 | 3 | 4 | 6 | | 8 | 9 | 10 | 12 | | |
| | | 0 | 10 | 20 | 30 | 40 | 50 | 60 | 70 | 80 | 90 | 100 |

**Fig. 19.** Subtest score profile of a patient with conduction aphasia.

for a cross: "Brazilian clothesbag"
for a thumb: "Argentine rifle"
for a metal ashtray: "beer-can thing"
for a necktie: "toenail . . . rusty nail"

Other examples of his jargon in extended utterances are, "He looks like he's up live walk . . . He looks like he's doing jack ofinarys . . . He lying wheaty. . . I don't know what you call that . . . He's taking souls."

The patient earned a severity rating of "1," as limited communication was possible through his partial comprehension of the examiner. (See Figure 20.) Inspection of the aphasia Subtest Summary Profile (Figure 21) reveals high fluency in relation to his severity rating, placing him unambiguously among the posterior aphasics. The rest of the profile shows elevated repetition, automatic speech, and paraphasia clusters in a context of minimal performance on all tests of propositional language, both oral and written. The tally of neologistic paraphasia, even though elevated, does not reflect his high propensity for these utterances, because the subtests were discontinued after his early failures, reducing the opportunity for paraphasias. His scores on the spatial-quantitative subtests are a series of total failures.

Inspection of the Profile of Speech Characteristics shows a configuration distinguishable by the high repetition rating from that of a classic Wernicke's aphasia. Only the high repetition and recitation scores on the aphasia examination reveal that this case is in the transcortical group. This is a case that illustrates the critical importance of repetition tests, and their evaluation in comparison to the level of other performances.

### Transcortical Motor Aphasia

(Luria—"Dynamic Aphasia.")

As in the preceding syndrome, the term, "transcortical," implies that repetition is particularly intact in a setting of otherwise limited speech.

The patient has great difficulty in initiating and organizing responses in conversation, unless the question is so highly structured that it can be answered with a one-word factual response. For example, when asked "What happened to you to bring you to the hospital?", the patient typically appears blocked and struggles with fragments such as "Well, I . . . it was . . . I can't." In contrast, if asked to name the day of the week, or the town he comes from, he responds promptly. By the same token, naming to confrontation is commonly well preserved. When these patients fail to retrieve a name on request, they respond remarkably well to prompting with the first sound.

It is common for patients with transcortical motor aphasia to break through occasionally with a fully grammatical and well-articulated sentence. Similarly, their ability to perform on repetition tasks is generally normal in articulation and grammar. While most often treated as "nonfluent" aphasics, the "fluency-nonfluency" dimension does not work well in this syndrome. The reader is reminded that "fluency" as a basis for categorizing aphasics is a pragmatic device that is useful in 80% or more of individuals. When a patient's output appears to straddle the two categories, it is quite meaningless to ask whether he is *really* a fluent or nonfluent aphasic.

The lesion producing transcortical motor aphasia is typically smaller than that for Broca's aphasia, occupying a zone just anterior or superior to the traditional Broca's area (the foot of the third frontal convolution), or in the subcortical region deep to Broca's area. In some instances, variants of the transcortical motor aphasia syndrome appear, which are characterized chiefly by relative superiority of repetition over spontaneous speech, but with more impairment of naming, auditory comprehension, and articulation than is observed in prototypical instances of this disorder.

On the Rating Scale Profile of Speech Characteristics, the features that are fairly constant are fair to good articulation, little or no paraphasia, a high repetition rating, and fair to excellent auditory comprehension. The ratings for Melodic Line, Phrase Length, Word Finding, and Grammatical Form may vary considerably, depending on how often the patient succeeds in producing well-formed phrases and sentences in his conversation. For those transcorticals who rarely have such breakthroughs, the ratings would be low; for the others the ratings could be high.

## APHASIA SEVERITY RATING SCALE

0.  No usable speech or auditory comprehension.

1.  All communication is through fragmentary expression; great need for inference, questioning, and guessing by the listener. The range of information that can be exchanged is limited, and the listener carries the burden of communication.

2.  Conversation about familiar subjects is possible with help from the listener. There are frequent failures to convey the idea, but patient shares the burden of communication with the examiner.

3.  The patient can discuss <u>almost all everyday problems</u> with little or no assistance. Reduction of speech and/or comprehension, however, makes conversation about certain material difficult or impossible.

4.  Some obvious loss of fluency in speech or facility of comprehension, without significant limitation on ideas expressed or form of expression.

5.  Minimal discernible speech handicaps; patient may have subjective difficulties that are not apparent to listener.

## RATING SCALE PROFILE OF SPEECH CHARACTERISTICS

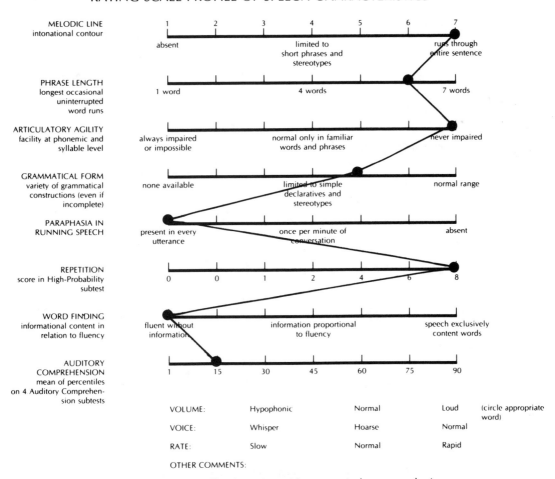

**Fig. 20.** Speech rating profile of a patient with transcortical sensory aphasia.

**SUBTEST SUMMARY PROFILE**

NAME: **C.N.**          DATE OF EXAM: **12-11-64**

| | PERCENTILES: | 0 | 10 | 20 | 30 | 40 | 50 | 60 | 70 | 80 | 90 | 100 |
|---|---|---|---|---|---|---|---|---|---|---|---|---|
| **SEVERITY RATING** | | | 0 | ⊛ | | | | 2 | | 3 | 4 | 5 |
| **FLUENCY** | ARTICULATION RATING | | 1 | 2 | 4 | 5 | 6 | | * | | | |
| | PHRASE LENGTH | | | 1 | 3 | 4 | 5 | * | 7 | | | |
| | MELODIC LINE | | 1 | 2 | 4 | | 6 | * | | | | |
| | VERBAL AGILITY (OMITTED) | | 0 | 2 | 5 | 6 | 8 | 9 | 11 | 13 | 14 | |
| **AUDITORY COMPREHENSION** | WORD DISCRIMINATION | 0 | 15 | 25 | 37 | 46 | 53 | 60 | 64 | 67 | 70 | 72 |
| | BODY-PART IDENTIFICATION | 0 | 1 | 5 | 10 | 13 | 15 | 16 | 17 | 18 | | 20 |
| | COMMANDS | 0 | 3 | 4 | 6 | 8 | 10 | 11 | 13 | 14 | 15 | |
| | COMPLEX IDEATIONAL MATERIAL | | | 2 | 3 | 4 | 5 | 6 | 8 | 9 | 11 | 12 |
| **NAMING** | RESPONSIVE NAMING | | | | 1 | 5 | 10 | 15 | 20 | 24 | 27 | 30 |
| | CONFRONTATION NAMING | | 0 | 9 | 28 | 43 | 60 | 72 | 84 | 94 | 105 | 114 |
| | ANIMAL NAMING | | | | | 1 | 2 | 3 | 4 | 6 | 9 | 23 |
| **ORAL READING** | WORD READING | | | | 1 | 3 | 7 | 15 | 21 | 26 | 30 | |
| | ORAL SENTENCE READING | | | | | | 1 | 2 | 4 | 7 | 9 | 10 |
| **REPETITION** | REPETITION OF WORDS | | 0 | 2 | 5 | 7 | 8 | | | | 10 | |
| | HIGH-PROBABILITY | | | 0 | 1 | | 2 | 4 | 5 | 7 | | |
| | LOW-PROBABILITY | | | | | 0 | 1 | | 2 | 4 | 6 | 8 |
| **PARAPHASIA** | NEOLOGISTIC | 40 | 16 | 9 | 4 | 2 | 1 | | 0 | | | |
| | LITERAL | 47 | 17 | 12 | 9 | 6 | 5 | 3 | | 1 | 0 | |
| | VERBAL | 40 | 23 | 18 | 15 | 12 | 9 | 7 | 4 | 3 | 1 | 0 |
| | EXTENDED | 75 | | 5 | 3 | 1 | 0 | | | | | |
| **AUTOMATIC SPEECH** | AUTOMATIZED SEQUENCES | | 0 | 1 | 2 | 3 | 4 | 6 | * | 8 | | |
| | RECITING | | | | 0 | 1 | | | * | | | |
| **READING COMPREHENSION** | SYMBOL DISCRIMINATION | 0 | 2 | 5 | 7 | 8 | 9 | | 10 | | | |
| | WORD RECOGNITION | 0 | 1 | 3 | 4 | 5 | 6 | 7 | | 8 | | |
| | COMPREHENSION OF ORAL SPELLING | | | | | 1 | | 3 | 4 | 6 | 7 | 8 |
| | WORD-PICTURE MATCHING | | 1 | | 4 | 6 | 8 | 9 | | 10 | | |
| | READING SENTENCES AND PARAGRAPHS | | 1 | 2 | 3 | 4 | 5 | 6 | 7 | 8 | | 10 |
| **WRITING** | MECHANICS | * | | 2 | | 3 | | 4 | | 5 | | |
| | SERIAL WRITING | | 7 | 18 | 25 | 30 | 33 | 40 | 43 | 46 | 47 | |
| | PRIMER-LEVEL DICTATION | | 1 | 4 | 6 | 9 | 11 | 13 | 14 | 15 | | |
| | SPELLING TO DICTATION | | | | | 1 | 2 | 3 | 5 | 7 | 10 | |
| | WRITTEN CONFRONTATION NAMING | | | 1 | 2 | 3 | 6 | 7 | 9 | 10 | | |
| | SENTENCES TO DICTATION | | | | 1 | 3 | 6 | 8 | 12 | | | |
| | NARRATIVE WRITING | | 1 | | | 2 | | | 3 | 4 | 5 | |
| **MUSIC** | SINGING | | 0 | 1 | | * | | | | | | |
| | RHYTHM | | 1 | | | | 2 | | | | | |
| **SPATIAL AND COMPUTATIONAL** | DRAWING TO COMMAND | 0 | 6 | 7 | 8 | 9 | 10 | 11 | 12 | | 13 | |
| | STICK MEMORY | 0 | 3 | 4 | 6 | 7 | 8 | 9 | 10 | 11 | 13 | 14 |
| | 3-D BLOCKS | | 0 | 2 | 4 | 5 | 6 | 7 | 8 | 9 | 10 | |
| | TOTAL FINGERS | 0 | 54 | 70 | 81 | 93 | 100 | 108 | 120 | 130 | 141 | 152 |
| | RIGHT-LEFT (OMITTED) | 0 | 1 | 3 | 4 | 6 | 8 | 9 | 11 | 14 | 16 | |
| | MAP ORIENTATION (OMITTED) | 0 | 2 | 5 | 6 | 9 | 11 | 13 | | 14 | | |
| | ARITHMETIC | | | 2 | 4 | 8 | 11 | 14 | 17 | 21 | 27 | 32 |
| | CLOCK SETTING | 0 | 3 | 4 | 6 | | 8 | 9 | 10 | 12 | | |
| | | 0 | 10 | 20 | 30 | 40 | 50 | 60 | 70 | 80 | 90 | 100 |

**Fig. 21.**  Score summary of a patient with transcortical sensory aphasia.

## Global Aphasia

In global aphasia, all aspects of language are so severely impaired that there is no longer a distinctive pattern of preserved versus impaired components. It is only articulation that is sometimes well preserved in the few words or stereotyped utterances that are preserved. Other patients with global aphasia may be totally unable to produce speech sounds voluntarily, even though they may utter an occasional word or short phrase as a spontaneous comment. It may be impossible to complete the Rating Scale Profile of Speech Characteristics for patients with global aphasia, if they do not produce enough speech to rate Melodic Line, Grammatical Form, or Word Finding.

Global aphasics sometimes produce stereotyped utterances that may consist of real or nonsense words. Some patients produce a continuous output of syllables that employ a limited set of vowel-consonant combinations and that make no sense, even though they are uttered with expressive intonation. As noted earlier, such output does not constitute paraphasia.

A few special observations on global aphasia are significant. Auditory comprehension of conversation concerning material of immediate personal relevance may appear fairly good in comparison to the patient's poor performance on all the formal auditory comprehension subtests. That is, the patient may indicate "yes" or "no" correctly and with assurance in response to questions about family members, current medical problems, or recent personal events in the hospital or at home. We have also found that many of these patients have a remarkably well-preserved ability to understand geographic place names and locate them on an outline map.

The lesion associated with global aphasia is usually a large one, encompassing both pre- and postrolandic speech zones.

## Mixed Nonfluent Aphasia

There is a border zone between Broca's aphasia and global aphasia for which we have coined the term "mixed nonfluent aphasia." This term is applied to patients who have the sparse output of Broca's aphasia, but whose auditory comprehension is too impaired for them to be assigned comfortably to the Broca category. While the designation of a cutoff is an arbitrary decision, we have used the fiftieth percentile in auditory comprehension as the point below which the term "mixed nonfluent" would be applied to patients who would otherwise be classified as Broca's aphasics. Since the mean auditory comprehension score of our global aphasics is at the fifteenth percentile with a standard deviation of about ten percentile points, severe nonfluent aphasics whose mean auditory comprehension score is below the twenty-fifth percentile are classified as global aphasics.

Patients falling into this category include partially recovered global aphasics who have recovered a degree of auditory comprehension and some ability to produce a few words and phrases.

## Subcortical Aphasias

Purely subcortical aphasia-producing lesions may be caused either by vascular occlusion or by intracerebral hemorrhage. Thromboses affecting the region of the internal capsule and putamen may vary considerably in size and in their posterior and superior extent. The corresponding variations in symptomatology are not yet clearly established.

Anterior subcortical aphasias involving the anterior limb of the internal capsule and putamen are characterized by sparse output with severely impaired articulation and hypophonic speech. Unlike patients with Broca's aphasia, those with subcortical lesions are not notably agrammatic. Extensive subcortical lesions that not only involve the putamen and anterior capsule but extend posteriorly to the neighborhood of the thalamus will produce a lasting global aphasia.

In contrast, several variants of fluent aphasia have been observed with posterior subcortical lesions, involving thalamus or neighboring white matter. These may closely resemble Wernicke's aphasia, but in some cases, both repetition and comprehension are spared, the major difficulties involving word finding and paraphasia. Unusually far-fetched paraphasic errors may intrude both in free conversation and in naming tasks. The latter pattern has been observed particularly in conjunction with hemorrhages of the thalamus or nearby areas (Alexander and LoVerme, 1980).

## Alexia with Agraphia

Patients with a lesion in the posterior margin of the language area, i.e., the angular gyrus, which bridges the posterior temporal and parietal regions, regularly present a defect in reading and writing, whereas speech and comprehension may be completely exempt from impairment.

In severe cases, the disturbance of reading may be so profound that the patient cannot match letters or words across styles of writing (upper to lower case, etc.), as tested by the Symbol and Word Discrimination subtest. More often, letter recognition is spared, and the patient can perform inconstantly with three- to four-letter primer words.

Writing is also severely impaired in that patients are unable to write letters from dictation or to transcribe from print into longhand, although slavish copying is usually preserved.

This syndrome may also occur in milder form with slow reading, spotted with misperceptions and failures to recognize even common words. In mild cases, elementary writing is preserved, but gross errors in spelling are common. In the effort of writing the patient loses track of the grammatical features and omits or misuses small words and inflectional endings, even though his oral speech is normal.

The anatomic localization of this syndrome in the angular gyrus usually brings along additional difficulties associated with this area. If speech is at all affected, the symptoms are those of a mild anomic aphasia. The complex of nonlanguage parietal lobe signs, however, is most reliably present to some degree. These include a marked difficulty in calculation, including clock-setting, finger identification, and right-left discrimination. The involvement of drawing and other visuospatial constructions is variable and may be quite severe. (For ex-amination procedures in the associated non-verbal defects, refer to Chapter 6.)

CONFIGURATION OF TEST SCORES. Since the patient with alexia and agraphia may have normal oral language, his Rating Scale Profile of Speech Characteristics may be indistinguishable from normal. The Subtest Summary Profile will show extremely low scores in the reading and writing clusters, however, and impairment in the spatial-quantitative tests.

## PURE APHASIAS

The "pure" aphasias have in common the feature of affecting only a single input or output modality, while leaving language virtually intact in all associated modalities. Pure aphasias are quite rare, especially pure agraphia.

## Aphemia

This disorder, which is also termed "subcortical motor aphasia," is an isolated disorder of articulation in which auditory comprehension, reading, and writing are intact. At first, the patient may be unable to produce any speech sounds, even in isolation, either in imitation or spontaneously, even failing automatic recitation, unlike Broca's aphasics. At this stage, the patient is truly anarthric, although he can phonate. The inability to imitate speech-like movements may or may not be paralleled by an apraxia for nonspeech oral movements.

As recovery takes place, articulation is painfully slow and awkward, but it is evident from the start that the patient speaks in grammatically complete sentences and has no word-finding difficulty.

Moreover, unlike the Broca's aphasic, whose articulation is facilitated by imitation or by the familiarity or automatic character of the utterance, the aphemic continues to show only a minimal relation between his articulatory difficulty and the linguistic nature of the speech content.

The supposed subcortical site to which the lesion is attributed makes logical sense in that it interrupts the final outflow of information from Broca's area to the speech effector system, without hampering cortical language activity.

## Pure Word Deafness

Almost as rare as pure agraphia is a condition in which auditory comprehension of language is lost without affecting speech output, reading, or writing. Patients with pure word deafness (also referred to as "subcortical sensory aphasia") react to sounds, but their response, when addressed, is similar to that of a deaf person. Unlike the Wernicke aphasic, they do not recognize speech as consisting of familiar acoustic patterns and are thus generally unable to repeat what they hear. Fragments of the message that do get through are in the form of sound elements, so that partial success in repeating is always a phonetic approximation, never a paraphasic association, as in Wernicke's aphasia.

On those occasions when a word is perceived and repeated, the patient at once understands it, demonstrating that, again unlike the case of Wernicke's aphasia, there is no dissociation of meaning from the acoustic pattern of the word.

While pure forms of this disorder are rare indeed, it is more often found with some of the features of Wernicke's aphasia, e.g., occasional paraphasic responses.

The anatomic associationistic model would suggest that the lesion for this disorder is one that destroys both the major primary auditory cortex (Heschl's gyrus) and the subcortical fibers, bringing information from the auditory association area of the minor hemisphere. Thus, in spite of a nearly intact Wernicke's area on the left, comprehension of speech is absent because no auditory input reaches this system, the adjacent auditory center being destroyed and the contralateral one isolated by interruption of transcallosal fibers. Wernicke's area continues to play its role in the production of speech and in reading and writing. In fact, however, the great majority of cases of pure word deafness have bilateral temporal lobe injury.

## Pure Alexia (Pure Word Blindness)

The least rare of the pure aphasias is alexia without agraphia—a most paradoxical disorder in which the patient can write normally but cannot read even his own handwriting. While a description of this disorder dating to 1588 is cited by Benton (1964), it was Déjerine (1892) who first provided the neuropathologic verification of the mechanism for this syndrome.

The patient with pure alexia is ordinarily blind in the right visual field of each eye, but has no visual perceptual problems in his normal field. His speech is normal, including the ability to name objects visually presented. Not only does he fail to read words, but even letters may be difficult or impossible; however, his comprehension of oral spelling is perfectly normal. By this means, he may use his limited ability to recognize individual letters to spell written words to himself and so achieve a laborious "reading." Number recognition is usually exempt from defect. Roman numerals, in spite of the fact that they are written with letters, are as well retained as arabic numbers.

A number of examiners of these patients report that they have an extraordinary difficulty in both naming and identifying colors from their spoken names, although they match and sort colors perfectly (Geschwind and Fusillo, 1966).

The usual lesion for this disorder is one that destroys the visual cortex of the left hemisphere and damages the splenium of the corpus callosum, the latter structure being essential for the communication between the two visual association areas. Thus, while the language area of the left hemisphere is undamaged, it is isolated from visual input. The ability to name objects may be spared because objects, unlike letters, arouse rich, multimodal sensory associations that are carried to the major hemisphere through other than the interrupted visual association pathways. In rare instances, visual object naming is also affected, as well as reading, resulting in "optic aphasia" (Freund, 1889).

## Pure Agraphia

The angular-gyrus-injured patient may suffer from a severe disorder of writing and spelling with only minimal involvement of reading. In these instances, as we have noted, other, nonverbal components of the angular gyrus syndrome are to be expected. A much rarer form of pure agraphia has been reported, attributed by Exner (1881) to a lesion of the foot of the second frontal convolution. This area lies in the motor association area and may represent a way station for the recoding of the output of Broca's area and/or the angular gyrus association areas into the form in which it can activate the effectors for writing movements. The rarity of pure agraphia is certainly due, at least in part, to the low probability of an isolated vascular lesion of the foot of the second frontal convolution. In addition, individual variation in the organization of the writing system may make only a few people susceptible to this disorder from a frontal lesion.

## CALLOSAL DISCONNECTION SYNDROMES

The partial isolation of the two hemispheres through injury or surgical section of the corpus callosum results in aphasic-like behavior related to the minor side of the body (i.e., the left side, in right-handed patients).

### Unilateral Tactile Aphasia

Tactile naming, on palpation of familiar objects with the eyes shut, is normally as easy with either hand as is naming to visual confrontation. Patients suffering from an interruption of callosal fibers may show a severe naming disorder only when palpating objects in the left hand, naming them promptly when the objects are transferred to the right hand. This unilateral anomia is not caused by lack of tactile recognition, because the patient can select from a multiple-choice array the object that he could not name, provided that the selection is performed with the left hand. He can draw the object with this left hand if it is not too complex (e.g., case of Geschwind and Kaplan, 1962).

Thus, while he "knows" what he has felt, this knowledge is confined to the nonspeaking right cerebral hemisphere. The right hand can neither draw nor select by touch what the left hand has felt.

### Unilateral Agraphia and Apraxia

On the expressive side, disconnection of the callosal pathways makes it impossible for the patient to write sensibly with the left hand, although he continues to do so normally with the right. Similarly, the callosal patient is unable to execute verbal commands involving the left limbs, whereas limb praxis to verbal command is intact on the right.

### Hemioptic Aphasia

When there has been a complete transection of the corpus callosum, extending to its posterior portion (splenium), objects experienced in the left visual field cannot be named, since no sensory information concerning them can reach the major hemisphere language area. Again, they can be picked out from multiple choice with the left hand, guided by the knowledge confined to the right side of the brain. This examination must ordinarily be conducted with a tachistoscopic arrangement in which the stimulus is flashed briefly to one side of the visual field to preclude scanning with both visual fields. No naturally occurring case of damage to both the splenium and anterior portions of the corpus callosum has been reported in which both visual fields were spared. Hemioptic aphasia has been described only in cases of surgical intervention for the control of bilaterally spreading epileptic discharges (Gazzaniga and Sperry, 1967).

# References

Alexander, M.P., and LoVerme, S.R.: Aphasia after left hemispheric subcortical hemorrhage. *Neurology, 30*:1193–1202, 1980.

Benson, D.F.: *Aphasia, Alexia and Agraphia.* New York, Churchill Livingstone, 1979.

Benton A.: Contributions to aphasia before Broca. *Cortex, 3*:314–329, 1964.

Borod, J., Goodglass, H., and Kaplan, E.: Normative data on the Boston Diagnostic Aphasia Examination, Parietal Lobe Battery and Boston Naming Test. *J. Clin. Neuropsychol., 2*:209–216, 1980.

Broca, P.: Perte de la parole. Ramollissement chronique et destruction partielle du lobe antérieur gauche du cerveau. *Bulletin de la Société d'anthropologie, II*:235–238, 1861.

Coltheart, M., Patterson, K., and Marshall, J.C.: *Deep Dyslexia.* London, Routledge and Kegan Paul, 1980.

Critchley, M.: *The Parietal Lobes.* New York, Hafner Publishing Company, 1966.

Damasio, H., and Damasio, A.R.: The anatomical basis of conduction aphasia. *Brain, 103*:337–350, 1980.

Déjerine, J.: "Des différentes variétés de cécité verbale." *Memoires de la Société Biologique,* 1892, Fév. 27, 1–30. Abstract in *Brain,* 1893, *16,* 318–320.

Eisenson, J.: *Examining for Aphasia.* New York, The Psychological Corporation, 1954.

Exner, S.: *Lokalisation des Funktion der Grosshirnrinde des Menschen.* Wien, Braunmuller, 1881.

Freund, C.S.: Uber optische Aphasie und Seelenblindheit. *Archiv. Psychiatrie Nervenkr., 20*:276–297, 371–416, 1889.

Gazzaniga, M., and Sperry, R.W.: "Language after section of the cerebral commissures." *Brain, 90*:131–148, 1967.

Gerstmann, J.: Syndrome of finger agnosia, disorientation for right and left, agraphia and acalculia. Arch. Neurol. Psychiatr., *44,*398–408, 1940.

Geschwind, N.: "Disconnexion syndromes in animals and man." *Brain.* 88:237–294, 585–644, 1965.

Geschwind, N.: "Carl Wernicke, the Breslau School and the history of aphasia." In E.C. Carterette, ed., *Brain function, III, Speech, Language and Communication,* U.C.L.A. Forum in the Medical Sciences, No. 4, University of California Press, pp. 1–16, 1966.

Geschwind, N.: The apraxias: Neural mechanisms of learned movement. *American Scientist, 63*:188–195, 1975.

Geschwind, N., and Fusillo, M.: "Color naming defects in association with alexia." *Archives of Neurology, 15*:137–146, 1966.

Geschwind, N., and Kaplan, E.: "A human cerebral deconnection syndrome." *Neurology, 12*:675, 685, 1962.

Geschwind, N., Segarra, J., and Quadfasel, F.A.: "Isolation of the speech area." *Neuropsychologia, 7*:327–340, 1968.

Goldstein, K.: *Language and Language Disturbance.* New York, Grune and Stratton, 1948.

Goldstein, K., and Scheerer, M.: *Abstract and Concrete Behavior.* Psychological Monographs, *53,* 329, 1941.

Goodglass, H., and Menn, L.: Is agrammatism a unitary phenomenon? *Agrammatism.* Edited by M.L. Kean. Academic Press, (in press).

Goodglass, H., Barton, M., and Kaplan, E.: "Sensory modality and object-naming in aphasia." *Journal of Speech and Hearing Research, 11*:488–496, 1968.

Goodglass H., Gleason J., and Hyde, M.: "Some dimensions of auditory language comprehension in aphasia." *Journal of Speech and Hearing Research, 13*:595–606, 1970.

Goodglass, H., and Kaplan, E.: "Disturbance of gesture and pantomime in aphasia." *Brain, 86,* 703–720, 1963.

Goodglass, H., Klein, H., Carey, P., and Jones, K.J.: "Specific semantic word categories in aphasia." *Cortex, 2*:74–89, 1966.

Goodglass, H., Quadfasel, F.A., and Timberlake, W.H.: "Phrase length and the type and severity of aphasia." *Cortex, 1*:133–153, 1964.

Head, H.: *Aphasia and Kindred Disorders of Speech.* New York, Macmillan, 1926.

Hécaen, H., and Dubois, J.: *Histoire de la Neuropsychologie du Langage.* Paris, Flammarion, 1969.

Heilman, K.M., and Valenstein, E. (Eds.): *Clinical Neuropsychology.* New York, Oxford University Press, 1979.

Kaplan, E.: *Gestural Representation of Implement Usage: An Organismic Developmental Study.* Doctoral dissertation, Clark University, 1968.

Lichtheim, L.: As cited in S. Freud. *On Aphasia.* New York, Universities Press, 1953.

Luria, A.R.: *Higher Cortical Functions in Man.* New York, Basic Books, 1966.

Luria, A.R.,: "Factors and forms of aphasia." In A.V.S. de Reuck and M. O'Connor, eds., *Disorders of Communication.* Boston, Little, Brown, 1964.

MacKay, D.G.: "Phonetic factors in the perception and recall of spelling errors." *Neuropsychologia, 6*:321–325, 1968.

Marshall, J.C., and Newcombe, F.: Patterns of paralexia: a psycholinguistic approach. *J. Psycholing. Res.,* 2:175–199, 1973.

McCarthy, J., and Kirk, S.A.: *Illinois Test of Psycholinguistic Abilities.* Urbana, University of Illinois, Institute of Research for Exceptional Children, 1966.

Miceli, G., Mazzucchi, A., Menn, L., and Goodglass, H.: Two contrasting cases of agrammatism in Italian. *Brain and Language, 19*:65–97, 1983.

Naeser, M.A., et al.: Aphasia with predominantly subcortical lesion sites. Arch. Neurol., *39*:2–14, 1982.

Schuell, H.: *Differential Diagnosis of Aphasia with the Minnesota Test.* Minneapolis, University of Minnesota Press, 1965.

Schuell, H., Jenkins, J.J., and Jiménez-Pabón, E.: *Aphasia in Adults.* New York, Harper and Row, 1964.

Spreen, O., Benton, A.L., and Van Allen, M.W.: "Dissociation of visual and tactile naming in amnesic aphasia." *Neurology, 16*:807–814, 1966.

Von Stockert, T., and Bader, L.: Some relations of grammar and lexicon. *Cortex, 12*:49–60, 1976.

Weisenburg, T.H., and McBride, K.E.: *Aphasia.* New York, Commonwealth Fund, 1935.

Wepman, J.M., and Jones, L.V.: *The Language Modalities Test for Aphasia.* Chicago, The Industrial Relations Center, University of Chicago, 1961.

# BOSTON DIAGNOSTIC APHASIA EXAMINATION BOOKLET

Lea & Febiger
200 Chester Field Parkway
Malvern, Pennsylvania   19355-9725
U.S.A.
(215) 251-2230
1-800-444-1785

# BOSTON DIAGNOSTIC APHASIA EXAMINATION

Date:

Patient:                                                        Case #:

Residence:

Age:                                                             Birthplace:

Date of birth:

Education:                                                     Grade completed:

                                                                     At what age?:

Occupational history:

Language background (circle one):          *English only*          *Bilingual*
    (If bilingual, brief language history)

Handedness history (including data on other family members):

Nature and duration of present illness:

Localizing information:

Hemiplegia (circle one):              *Right*        *Left*        *Recovered*        *Absent*

Hemianopsia (circle one):            *Right*        *Left*        *Recovered*        *Absent*

EEG Focus:

Operative information:

Other localizing information (e.g., scan findings, arteriogram, etc.):

# I. CONVERSATIONAL AND EXPOSITORY SPEECH

Conduct informal exchange, incorporating suggested questions, to elicit as many of the desired responses as possible. Record verbatim. Tape record, if possible.

a. Response to greeting. (Q. "HOW ARE YOU TODAY?" or equivalent):

b. Response with "yes" or "no." (Q. "HAVE YOU EVER BEEN IN THIS HOSPITAL BEFORE?" or "HAVE I TESTED YOU BEFORE?"):

c. Response with "I think so," or equivalent. (Q. "DO YOU THINK WE CAN HELP YOU?" or ". . . HAVE HELPED YOU?"):

d. Response with "I don't know" or equivalent. (Q. "WHEN ARE YOUR TREATMENTS GOING TO BE FINISHED?"):

e. Response with "I hope so" or equivalent. (Q. "BEFORE TOO LONG LET'S HOPE. WHAT DO YOU SAY?"):

f. "What is your full name?":

g. "What is your full address?" (Accept as correct any response that includes street and number or street and city.):

h. *Open-ended conversation:* In order to elicit as much free conversation as possible, it is suggested that examiner start with familiar topics such as, "What kind of work were you doing before you became ill?" and "Tell me what happened to bring you to the hospital." Encourage patient to speak for at least *10 minutes,* if possible. (Minimize use of "yes"-"no" questions and probing for specific facts.) If tape recording is not used, record as much as possible verbatim.

i. Presentation of picture. Show the test picture and tell patient: "Tell everything you see going on in this picture." Point to neglected features of the picture and ask for elaboration if patient's response is skimpier than his apparent potential. A minute is usually enough time.

Cookie Theft (Card 1)

# II. AUDITORY COMPREHENSION

## A. *Word Discrimination*

Present test Cards 2 and 3 separately. Have patient look over all pictures on the card presented before starting. Then ask him to point out each picture or symbol by saying, "Show me the _____." Rotate at random from one category to another. One repetition is permitted, on request. If the patient does not find the correct category, then show him the category, to the exclusion of the others, and repeat the name of the item to be identified. (Score in the "CUE" column.) Correct discrimination ("identification") is scored 2 points if within 5 seconds, 1 point otherwise. Attention to the correct category without correct discrimination is scored ½ point (check CATEGORY).

| Card 2 | IDENTIFICATION | | CATE-GORY | CUE | FAIL | Card 3 | IDENTIFICATION | | CATE-GORY | CUE | FAIL |
|---|---|---|---|---|---|---|---|---|---|---|---|
| | Under 5 seconds | Over 5 seconds | 1/2 | 1/2 | | | Under 5 seconds | Over 5 seconds | 1/2 | 1/2 | |
| OBJECTS: | 2 points | 1 point | point | point | 0 | ACTIONS: | 2 points | 1 point | point | point | 0 |
| chair | | | | | | smoking | | | | | |
| key | | | | | | drinking | | | | | |
| glove | | | | | | running | | | | | |
| feather | | | | | | sleeping | | | | | |
| hammock | | | | | | falling | | | | | |
| cactus | | | | | | dripping | | | | | |
| LETTERS: | | | | | | COLORS: | | | | | |
| L | | | | | | blue | | | | | |
| H | | | | | | brown | | | | | |
| R | | | | | | red | | | | | |
| T | | | | | | pink | | | | | |
| S | | | | | | gray | | | | | |
| G | | | | | | purple | | | | | |
| FORMS: | | | | | | NUMBERS: | | | | | |
| circle | | | | | | 7 | | | | | |
| spiral | | | | | | 42 | | | | | |
| square | | | | | | 700 | | | | | |
| triangle | | | | | | 1936 | | | | | |
| cone | | | | | | 15 | | | | | |
| star | | | | | | 7000 | | | | | |

Raw Score: [    ]

## B. *Body-Part Identification*

Ask patient to point to the following body parts. Record incorrect responses.

*Scoring:* Items in the first 2 columns are scored 1 point if recognized promptly (within approximately 5 seconds) and ½ point if identified correctly, but after hesitation. The third column is for right-left discrimination and receives a total of 2 points if all 8 are correct (the body part may be incorrect as long as right-left discrimination is made), 1 point if 6 or 7 items are correct, otherwise 0.

| | BODY-PART IDENTIFICATION | | | | | | | | | RIGHT-LEFT DISCRIMINATION | | |
|---|---|---|---|---|---|---|---|---|---|---|---|---|
| | Correct | | Fail | | | Correct | | Fail | | | Correct | Failed |
| | <5" | >5" | | | | <5" | >5" | | | | | |
| | 1 point | ½ point | | | | 1 point | ½ point | | | | | |
| ear | | | | | wrist | | | | | right ear | | |
| nose | | | | | thumb | | | | | left shoulder | | |
| shoulder | | | | | thigh | | | | | left knee | | |
| knee | | | | | chin | | | | | right ankle | | |
| eyelid | | | | | elbow | | | | | right wrist | | |
| ankle | | | | | lips | | | | | left thumb | | |
| chest | | | | | eyebrow | | | | | right elbow | | |
| neck | | | | | cheek | | | | | left cheek | | |
| middle finger | | | | | index finger | | | | | 8 correct<br>6 7 correct | 2 points<br>1 point | |

**Raw Score:** ☐

## C. *Commands*

Have the patient carry out the following commands, giving credit for each underlined element that he carries out. One repetition is permitted on request, but command must always be repeated as a whole, not broken up.

1. Make a *fist.*
2. Point to the *ceiling,* then to the *floor.*
   (After lining up a pencil, watch, and card, in that order, on the table before the patient.)
3. Put the *pencil on top of the card,* then *put it back.*
4. Put the *watch* on the *other side of the pencil* and *turn over* the *card.*
5. Tap *each shoulder twice* with *two fingers* keeping your *eyes shut.*

**Raw Score:** ☐

( 7 )

## D. *Complex Ideational Material*

The only response required is either agreement or disagreement. Both the "a" and the "b" questions for each numbered item must be answered correctly to receive credit of one point. One repetition of each question is permitted.

| | |
|---|---|
| Will a cork sink in water? | 1a |
| Is a hammer good for cutting wood? | 2a |
| Do two pounds of flour weigh more than one? | 3a |
| Will water go through a good pair of rubber boots? | 4a |
| Will a stone sink in water? | 1b |
| Can you use a hammer to pound nails? | 2b |
| Is one pound of flour heavier than two? | 3b |
| Will a good pair of rubber boots keep water out? | 4b |

"I am going to read you a short story and then I will ask you some questions about it. Are you ready?"   (Read at a normal rate.)

Mr. Jones had to go to New York. He decided to take a train. His wife drove him to the station but on the way they had a flat tire. However, they arrived at the station just in time for him to catch the train.

| | |
|---|---|
| Did Mr. Jones miss his train? | 5a |
| Was Mr. Jones going to New York? | 6a |
| Did he get to the station on time? | 5b |
| Was he on his way home from New York? | 6b |

"I am going to read another paragraph. Are you ready?"

A soldier tried to cash a check in a bank near his camp. The teller, firm but sympathetic, said, "You will have to have identification from some of your friends from the camp." The discouraged soldier answered, "But I don't have any friends in camp—I'm the bugler."

| | |
|---|---|
| Was the soldier's check cashed at once? | 7a |
| Did the soldier have a friend with him? | 8a |
| Did the teller object to cashing the check? | 7b |
| Did the soldier have trouble finding friends? | 8b |

( 8 )

I will read another one. Are you ready?"

A customer walked into a hotel carrying a coil of rope in one hand and a suitcase in the other. The hotel clerk asked, "Pardon me, sir, but will you tell me what the rope is for?"
"Yes," responded the man, "that's my fire escape!"
"I'm sorry, sir," said the clerk, "but all guests carrying their own fire escapes must pay in advance."

Was the customer carrying a suitcase in each hand?          9a

Was the clerk suspicious of this guest?                              10a

Was he carrying something unusual in one hand?          9b

Did the clerk trust this guest?                                          10b

"I am going to read one more paragraph. Listen carefully."

The lion cub is born with a deep-seated hunting instinct. One cub will stalk and pounce on another with the same eagerness and thrill exhibited by a kitten. During the year and a half of cubhood this play develops into a hunting and killing technique. Skill comes through long practice, imitation of the old lions and obedience to warning growls of the mother.

Does this paragraph tell how lions learn to hunt?          11a

Does this paragraph say lions are skillful killers          12a
from the time they are born?

Does it tell how to hunt lions?                                          11b

Does it say lions need practice before they can          12b
kill their prey?

**Raw Score:** ☐

( 9 )

# III. ORAL EXPRESSION

## A. *Oral Agility*

1. *Nonverbal agility:* Have the patient carry out the following rapidly repeated mouth movements as well as he can, after you demonstrate and describe the movement.

Count the number of full alternations carried out in 5 seconds.

2. *Verbal agility:* Have the patient repeat the following words as rapidly as he can, while you time the number of repetitions for 5 seconds. Any assistance that helps patient to produce the desired word initially is permitted.* Use printed words on Card 4.

| Action Required | Number of times in 5"  2 points | 1 point |
|---|---|---|
| a. Purse lips, release | 8 | 4–7 |
| b. Open and close mouth | 10 | 6–9 |
| c. Retract lips, release | 8 | 4–7 |
| d. Tongue to alternate corners of mouth | 8 | 4–7 |
| e. Protrude and retract tongue | 8 | 4–7 |
| f. Tongue to upper and lower teeth | 7 | 3–6 |

| Test Words | Number of times in 5"  2 points | 1 point |
|---|---|---|
| a. Mama, mama . . . etc. | 9 | 3–8 |
| b. Tip-top, tip-top | 6 | 2–5 |
| c. Fifty-fifty, fifty-fifty | 5 | 2–4 |
| d. Thanks, thanks | 9 | 3–8 |
| e. Huckleberry, huckleberry | 7 | 3–6 |
| f. Baseball player, baseball player | 5 | 2–4 |
| g. Caterpillar, caterpillar | 7 | 3–6 |

Raw Score: ☐

Raw Score: ☐

*If patient cannot get started on *one or two items at the most,* either because of perseveration or paraphasic substitution, eliminate items and prorate score (7/5 or 7/6, as appropriate, to nearest whole number). If more than two items are unscoreable, do not enter total score.

## Scoring of Articulation Ratings and Paraphasias

Subtests B and D through H provide for the recording of paraphasic responses and for the assignment of an articulation rating of Normal, Stiff, Distorted, and Failed for each response that is a recognizable attempt at the target word and is not paraphasic. Definitions for these articulation ratings will be found on page 36 of Assessment of Aphasia and Related Disorders, 1983 (or pages 30 to 31 of the 1972 edition).

Articulation ratings are recorded for the examiner's guidance in reviewing the test protocol, and ratings of Normal, Stiff, or Distorted all denote that the response is scored as correct. A response is scored as a failure if it is rated as Failed in articulation, or if an uncorrected paraphasia or no response is given.

Paraphasias are to be entered in their respective columns (see p. 11 of this booklet) and counted in the tally of paraphasias even when they are self-corrected. Credit for the item is then allowed, even though the paraphasia is counted.

Paraphasic errors in single words.

1. *Neologistic distortion*—more than half of the sounds produced are extraneous to the desired word. This term applies only to responses that are spoken as a unit with some fluency of articulation. It does not apply to sounds produced awkwardly by subjects groping for the correct articulatory position. The latter responses would simply be scored as failures or as severely distorted in articulation if the word is recognizable.

2. *Literal paraphasia*—response contains sounds or syllables that have slipped out of sequence, have been deleted, or are entirely extraneous to the desired response, but more than half of the response corresponds to more than half of the required word.

3. *Verbal paraphasia*—substitution of an inappropriate word during the effort to say something specific.

Paraphasic errors in connected speech (Extended Paraphasia).

4. *Other*—this category applies to a number of types of paraphasia involving more than a single word and to some nonparaphasic responses. Examiner should write in an abbreviation of a category rather than use a checkmark only.

*pg*    paragrammatism—well-articulated, connected utterance composed of real words in a semantically unacceptable form ("extended English jargon" in first edition)

*npg*   neologistic paragrammatism—well-articulated, connected utterance composed largely of neologisms interspersed with some normal grammatical morphemes ("extended neologistic jargon" in 1972 edition)

*cl*    circumlocution

*irrel* irrelevant comment, normal in syntax

Note: Recurring syllables or real words from a small stereotyped repertoire are *not* scored as paraphasia. Similarly, continuous mumbling or output of syllables that are not segmented into "words" is not scored as paraphasia.

## B. *Automatized Sequences*

Have patient recite each of the following four series, giving him assistance with the first word, if necessary. Provide further assistance as needed, but discontinue a series when patient fails with four successive words. Record assistance given by circling the word; cross out words omitted by patient. Allow 0, 1, or 2 points, as indicated.

| ARTICULATION | | | | | | | PARAPHASIA | | | |
|---|---|---|---|---|---|---|---|---|---|---|
| Normal | Stiff | Distorted | Fail | | 1 point | 2 points | Neologistic Distortion | Literal | Verbal | Other |
| | | | | **1.** *Days of the week:* | | | | | | |
| ⋯ | ⋯ | ⋯ | ⋯ | Sun.  Mon.  Tues. | | | ⋯ | ⋯ | ⋯ | ⋯ |
| ⋯ | ⋯ | ⋯ | ⋯ | Wed.  Thur.  Fri.  Sat. | 4 consecutive | all | ⋯ | ⋯ | ⋯ | ⋯ |
| | | | | **2.** *Months of the year:* | | | | | | |
| ⋯ | ⋯ | ⋯ | ⋯ | Jan.  Feb.  Mar.  April | | | ⋯ | ⋯ | ⋯ | ⋯ |
| ⋯ | ⋯ | ⋯ | ⋯ | May  June  July  Aug. | | | ⋯ | ⋯ | ⋯ | ⋯ |
| ⋯ | ⋯ | ⋯ | ⋯ | Sept.  Oct.  Nov.  Dec. | 5 consecutive | all | ⋯ | ⋯ | ⋯ | ⋯ |
| | | | | **3.** *Counting to 21:* | | | | | | |
| ⋯ | ⋯ | ⋯ | ⋯ | 1  2  3  4  5  6  7  8  9 | | | ⋯ | ⋯ | ⋯ | ⋯ |
| ⋯ | ⋯ | ⋯ | ⋯ | 10  11  12  13  14  15  16 | | | ⋯ | ⋯ | ⋯ | ⋯ |
| ⋯ | ⋯ | ⋯ | ⋯ | 17  18  19  20  21 | 8 consecutive | all | ⋯ | ⋯ | ⋯ | ⋯ |
| | | | | **4.** *Alphabet:* | | | | | | |
| ⋯ | ⋯ | ⋯ | ⋯ | a  b  c  d  e  f  g  h | | | ⋯ | ⋯ | ⋯ | ⋯ |
| ⋯ | ⋯ | ⋯ | ⋯ | i  j  k  l  m  n  o  p  q | | | ⋯ | ⋯ | ⋯ | ⋯ |
| ⋯ | ⋯ | ⋯ | ⋯ | r  s  t  u  v  w  x  y  z | 7 consecutive | all | ⋯ | ⋯ | ⋯ | ⋯ |

**Raw Score:** ☐

## C. Recitation, Singing, and Rhythm

Instruct patient to complete the line for the following rhymes. Words in parentheses may be given as additional cues, if necessary. Use a natural or slightly exaggerated inflection to encourage completion of the rhyme. If patient fails, or is not familiar with the material, attempt other memorized or automatized material, such as the Lord's Prayer, the Pledge of Allegiance, etc. Circle qualitative ratings below.

1. *Reciting:*

   Jack and Jill (went) . . . . . . . . . .   There was an old woman who lived in a
   shoe, (she had) . . . . . . . . . . . . . . . . . . . . .

   Baa, Baa, black sheep (have) . .
   My country ('tis) . . . . . . . . . . . . . . . . . . . .

   Hickory dickory dock   (Sweet) . . . . . . . . . . . . . . . . . . . . . . . . . . . .
   (The mouse) . . . . . . . . . . . . . . . . .   (Of thee) . . . . . . . . . . . . . . . . . . . . . . . .

2. *Singing:* After recitation of "My Country 'Tis of Thee," have patient sing this or any other song with which he is familiar.

3. *Rhythm:* Examiner taps out the following rhythms on the desk in continuous fashion (6 times) until the patient demonstrates that he can or cannot repeat tempo.

   $\smile$ ' $\smile$ ' (repeat) (as in: "along, along")
   ' $\smile$ $\smile$ ' $\smile$ $\smile$ (repeat) (as in: "Longfellow")
   $\smile$ ' ' $\smile$ ' ' (repeat) (as in: "a long time")
   ' $\smile$ $\smile$ ' ',' ' (as in: "Shave and a haircut, two bits")

RATINGS:          *Reciting*          *Singing*          *Rhythm*
                                      (Melody)

2 = Good
1 = Impaired
0 = Failed

## D. *Repetition of Words*

Have patient repeat each of the following words. One repetition by examiner is permitted when it appears that this may help, or when it is requested. For credit, all syllables must be in their proper order, although distortion of individual sound elements is permitted, provided that it is in keeping with patient's general articulation difficulty and that the word is recognizable.

| ARTICULATION | | | | | PARAPHASIA | | | |
|---|---|---|---|---|---|---|---|---|
| Normal | Stiff | Distorted | Fail | | Neolo-gistic | Literal | Verbal | Other |
| | | | | brown | | | | |
| | | | | chair | | | | |
| | | | | what | | | | |
| | | | | hammock | | | | |
| | | | | purple | | | | |
| | | | | W | | | | |
| | | | | fifteen | | | | |
| | | | | 1776 | | | | |
| | | | | emphasize | | | | |
| | | | | Methodist Episcopal | | | | |

**Raw Score:** ☐

## E. Repeating Phrases

Have patient repeat the following phrases. Alternate between columns 1 and 2. On patient's request, a single repetition of the entire test phrase is permitted without loss of credit.

| ARTICULATION | | | | | | PARAPHASIA | | | |
|---|---|---|---|---|---|---|---|---|---|
| Normal | Stiff | Distorted | Fail | 1. High Probability / 2. Low Probability | | Neologistic Distortion | Literal | Verbal | Other |
| | | | | a. You know how. | | | | | |
| | | | | | a. The vat leaks. | | | | |
| | | | | b. Down to earth. | | | | | |
| | | | | | b. Limes are sour. | | | | |
| | | | | c. I got home from work. | | | | | |
| | | | | | c. The spy fled to Greece. | | | | |
| | | | | d. You should not tell her. | | | | | |
| | | | | | d. Pry the tin lid off. | | | | |
| | | | | e. Go ahead and do it if possible. | | | | | |
| | | | | | e. The Chinese fan had a rare emerald. | | | | |
| | | | | f. Near the table in the dining room. | | | | | |
| | | | | | f. The barn swallow captured a plump worm. | | | | |
| | | | | g. They heard him speak on the radio last night. | | | | | |
| | | | | | g. The lawyer's closing argument convinced him. | | | | |
| | | | | h. I stopped at his front door and rang the bell. | | | | | |
| | | | | | h. The phantom soared across the foggy heath. | | | | |

**High-Probability Raw Score:** ☐

**Low-Probability Raw Score:** ☐

( 15 )

## F. Word Reading

Have the patient read the words, one at a time, from test Card 5. Check approximate lag between your pointing to the word and the patient's adequate response. Assist as required, but give no credit for responses obtained with help.

| ARTICULATION | | | | | Approximate response lag | | | | PARAPHASIA | | | |
| Normal | Stiff | Distorted | Fail | Test Words | 0–3″ 3 points | 3–10″ 2 points | 10–30″ 1 point | Fail 0 | Neol. Dist. | Literal | Verbal | Other |
|---|---|---|---|---|---|---|---|---|---|---|---|---|
| | | | | chair | | | | | | | | |
| | | | | circle | | | | | | | | |
| | | | | hammock | | | | | | | | |
| | | | | triangle | | | | | | | | |
| | | | | fifteen | | | | | | | | |
| | | | | purple | | | | | | | | |
| | | | | seven-twenty-one | | | | | | | | |
| | | | | dripping | | | | | | | | |
| | | | | brown | | | | | | | | |
| | | | | smoking | | | | | | | | |

Raw Score: ☐

## G. Responsive Naming

Have patient supply the one-word responses required by the stimulus questions. Check approximate lag.

| ARTICULATION | | | | | Approximate response lag | | | | PARAPHASIA | | | |
| Normal | Stiff | Distorted | Fail | Question | 0–3″ 3 points | 3–10″ 2 points | 10–30″ 1 point | Fail 0 | Neol. Dist. | Literal | Verbal | Other |
|---|---|---|---|---|---|---|---|---|---|---|---|---|
| | | | | What do we tell time with? | | | | | | | | |
| | | | | What do you do with a razor? | | | | | | | | |
| | | | | What do you do with soap? | | | | | | | | |
| | | | | What do you do with a pencil? | | | | | | | | |
| | | | | What do we cut paper with? | | | | | | | | |
| | | | | What color is grass? | | | | | | | | |
| | | | | What do we light a cigarette with? | | | | | | | | |
| | | | | How many things in a dozen? | | | | | | | | |
| | | | | What color is coal? | | | | | | | | |
| | | | | Where do you go to buy medicine? | | | | | | | | |

Raw Score: ☐

( 16 )

## H. *Visual Confrontation Naming*

Have the patient name each item in the order listed as you point to it on Cards 2 and 3. Assist, if necessary, to preserve rapport, but do not credit responses so obtained. Check under column that indicates appropriate lag in giving response, and score accordingly. Articulation and paraphasia should be rated wherever possible.

| ARTICULATION | | | | | Approximate response lag | | | | PARAPHASIA | | | |
| Normal | Stiff | Distorted | Fail | Test Items | 0–3″ 3 points | 3–10″ 2 points | 10–30″ 1 point | Fail 0 | Neologistic Distortion | Literal | Verbal | Other |
|---|---|---|---|---|---|---|---|---|---|---|---|---|
| | | | | *Objects:* chair | | | | | | | | |
| | | | | key | | | | | | | | |
| | | | | glove | | | | | | | | |
| | | | | feather | | | | | | | | |
| | | | | hammock | | | | | | | | |
| | | | | cactus | | | | | | | | |
| | | | | *Letters:* H | | | | | | | | |
| | | | | T | | | | | | | | |
| | | | | R | | | | | | | | |
| | | | | L | | | | | | | | |
| | | | | S | | | | | | | | |
| | | | | G | | | | | | | | |
| | | | | *Geometric Forms:* square | | | | | | | | |
| | | | | triangle | | | | | | | | |
| | | | | *Actions:* running | | | | | | | | |
| | | | | sleeping | | | | | | | | |
| | | | | drinking | | | | | | | | |
| | | | | smoking | | | | | | | | |
| | | | | falling | | | | | | | | |
| | | | | dripping | | | | | | | | |
| | | | | *Numbers:* 7 | | | | | | | | |
| | | | | 15 | | | | | | | | |
| | | | | 700 | | | | | | | | |
| | | | | 1936 | | | | | | | | |
| | | | | 42 | | | | | | | | |
| | | | | 7000 | | | | | | | | |
| | | | | *Colors:* red | | | | | | | | |
| | | | | brown | | | | | | | | |
| | | | | pink | | | | | | | | |
| | | | | blue | | | | | | | | |
| | | | | gray | | | | | | | | |
| | | | | purple | | | | | | | | |
| | | | | *Body parts:* ear | | | | | | | | |
| | | | | nose | | | | | | | | |
| | | | | elbow | | | | | | | | |
| | | | | shoulder | | | | | | | | |
| | | | | ankle | | | | | | | | |
| | | | | wrist | | | | | | | | |

**Raw Score:** ☐

J. *Animal Naming (Fluency in Controlled Association)*

Instruct the patient: "I want to see how many different animals you can call to mind and name for about a minute, while I count them. Any animals will do; they can be from the farm, the jungle, the ocean or house pets. For instance you can start with dog." Start timing from this point and continue for a minute and a half. Score is based on the most productive consecutive 60 seconds. Record verbatim below.

First 15″        15–30″        30–45″        45–60″        60–75″        75–90″

Raw Score: ☐

## K. *Oral Sentence Reading*

Have the patient read the following sentences aloud from test Cards 6 and 7. Indicate by marking on this record any assistance given, omissions, substitutions, etc. One point credit is allowed for each completely correct sentence.

| | Correct 1 point | Fail |
|---|---|---|
| You know how. | | |
| Down to earth. | | |
| I got home from work. | | |
| Near the table in the dining room. | | |
| They heard him speak on the radio last night. | | |
| Limes are sour. | | |
| The spy fled to Greece. | | |
| The barn swallow captured a plump worm. | | |
| The lawyer's closing argument convinced him. | | |
| The phantom soared across the foggy heath. | | |

**Raw Score:** ⬜

# IV. UNDERSTANDING WRITTEN LANGUAGE

A. *Symbol and Word Discrimination*

Point to the model letter or word on Cards 8 and 9 and have the patient locate the correct corresponding word or letter in the row beneath it.

| | | | |
|---|---|---|---|
| on | _____ | dog | _____ |
| G | _____ | B | _____ |
| H | _____ | who | _____ |
| was | _____ | F | _____ |
| K | _____ | pal | _____ |

**Raw Score:** [    ]

B. *Phonetic Association*

1. *Word recognition:*

Have patient point out the written word on Cards 10 and 11 corresponding to the one you give orally. The patient should be guided to the correct line on the test card. Use the following eight oral test words.

| | | | |
|---|---|---|---|
| ship | _____ | puppy | _____ |
| pond | _____ | drizzle | _____ |
| book | _____ | hollow | _____ |
| with | _____ | explode | _____ |

**Raw Score:** [    ]

2. *Comprehension of oral spelling:*

Spell the following words for the patient and have him orally identify the spelled word.

| | |
|---|---|
| N-O | B-R-O-W-N |
| M-A-N | E-L-B-O-W |
| G-I-R-L | F-I-F-T-E-E-N |
| W-H-I-P | W-H-I-S-K-E-Y |

**Raw Score:** [    ]

C. *Word-Picture Matching*

Using Cards 2 and 3, and Card 5, have patient pick out appropriate picture for each word shown him. ("Which of these pictures is this word?") Discourage patients from reading aloud.

| | | | |
|---|---|---|---|
| chair | _____ | purple | _____ |
| circle | _____ | seven-twenty-one | _____ |
| hammock | _____ | dripping | _____ |
| triangle | _____ | brown | _____ |
| fifteen | _____ | smoking | _____ |

**Raw Score:** ☐

D. *Reading Sentences and Paragraphs*

Patient is presented with Cards 12, 13, 14, 15, and 16 successively. Patient indicates his selection on the card, and the examiner underlines the choice in the test booklet. Assistance may be given in the two examples, but not in the test proper.

*EXAMPLES*

WATER IS _____    CHILDREN PLAY _____

FLY    WET    DRY    RED        DOOR    SHOE    DIME    BALL

1. A DOG CAN _____

     TALK          BARK          SING          CAT

2. A MOTHER HAS A _____

     TREE          COOK          CHILD          TRUCK

3. MR. JONES GIVES HAIRCUTS AND SHAMPOOS. HE IS A _____

     SHAVING          BOY          BUTCHER          BARBER

4. MANY BIRDS COME BACK IN THE SUMMER. THEY BUILD _____

     NESTS          EGGS          SPARROW          CAT

5. SCHOOLS AND ROADS COST MONEY. WE ALL PAY FOR THEM THROUGH _____
   HOUSES          COUNTRY          TAXES          POLICE

6. ARTISTS ARE PEOPLE WHO MAKE BEAUTIFUL PAINTINGS OR STATUES. ANOTHER KIND OF ARTIST IS A _____

   PICTURE          MUSICIAN          LIBRARY          SOLDIER

7. ALUMINUM WAS ONCE VERY COSTLY TO REFINE. NOW, ELECTRICITY HAS SOLVED THE RE-FINING PROBLEM, AND ALUMINUM HAS BECOME _____

   VERY STRONG      MUCH CHEAPER      A MINER          ELECTRONIC

8. THE CONNECTION BETWEEN SANITATION AND DISEASE BECAME CLEAR WHEN PASTEUR SHOWED THAT FOOD WOULD NOT DECAY IF GERMS WERE KILLED BY HEAT AND THEN SEALED OUT. STERILIZATION BY HEAT IS A RESULT OF _____

   SANITATION       GOOD FOOD         PASTEUR'S DISCOVERY       GERMS

9. FAVORITISM USED TO BE THE RULE IN CIVIL SERVICE, AND MANY JOBS PAID MORE THAN THEY WERE WORTH. CIVIL SERVICE REFORM HAS RESULTED IN CLASSIFYING POSITIONS ACCORDING TO THEIR DUTIES AND RESPONSIBILITIES. THE AIM OF CIVIL SERVICE CLASSI-FICATION IS TO _____

   ACHIEVE HIGHER SALARIES          ESTABLISH FAVORITISM

   EFFECT A REDUCTION IN TAXES      ASSURE EQUAL PAY FOR EQUAL WORK

10. IN THE EARLY DAYS OF THIS COUNTRY, THE FUNCTIONS OF GOVERNMENT WERE FEW IN NUMBER. MOST OF THESE FUNCTIONS WERE CARRIED OUT BY LOCAL TOWN AND COUNTY OFFICIALS, WHILE CENTRALIZED AUTHORITY WAS DISTRUSTED. THE GROWTH OF INDUSTRY AND OF BIG CITIES HAS SO CHANGED THE SITUATION THAT THE FARMER OF TODAY IS CONCERNED WITH _____

   LOCAL AFFAIRS ABOVE ALL          THE PRICE OF LUMBER

   THE ACTIONS OF THE GOVERNMENT    THE AUTHORITY OF TOWN OFFICIALS

**Raw Score:** ⬜

# V. WRITING

A. *Mechanics of Writing*

Recall and execution of writing movements. Have the patient execute the following (use top section of page 24 or unlined paper):

1. Name and address

2. If (1) is failed then print the patient's name and address on the paper and have him copy it.

3. Transcribe: Have the patient transcribe the sentence printed in the middle of page 24. (Note: Have the patient *write* directly on the page below the sentence. If patient cannot transcribe into longhand, have him copy in block printing.)

Evaluation of mechanics of writing is based on inspection of patient's entire written output in the writing section. Use the five-level scale listed here.

1. No legible letters.

2. Occasional success on single letters (block printing).

3. Block printing with some malformed letters.

4. Legible but impaired cursive writing and/or upper- and lower-case printing.

5. Judged to be the same as premorbid writing, with allowance made for use of nonpreferred hand.

*Mechanics Rating:* _____

B. *Recall of Written Symbols*

For all writing tasks, continue on page 24 if practical or use additional sheets of unlined paper as necessary. Have the patient write the following:

1. *Serial writing*          Letters correct: _____

    alphabet (26 points)      Numbers correct: _____

    numbers through 21 (21 points)    Letters plus numbers: _____

                                     **Raw Score:** ☐

2. *Primer-level dictation.* Dictate the following:

    a. Single letters:           Circle number correct:

      B–K–L–R–T         0  1  2  3  4  5

    b. Numbers:

      7–15–42–193–1865      0  1  2  3  4  5

    c. Primary words:

      GO–BOY–RUN–COME–BABY    0  1  2  3  4  5

                                       **Raw Score:** ☐

( 23 )

THE QUICK BROWN FOX JUMPS OVER THE LAZY DOG

C. *Written Word-Finding*

1. *Spelling to dictation:* Give the following words orally and ask the patient to write them. If a word is failed (spelled incorrectly or not written at all), have the patient spell the word orally and record in appropriate column. Oral spelling is not entered in the score summary data.

|  | *Written* | *Oral* |  |
|---|---|---|---|
| SOFT | _____ | _____ | |
| BELONG | _____ | _____ | |
| SOAP | _____ | _____ | |
| FIGHT | _____ | _____ | |
| UNCLE | _____ | _____ | |
| LIBERTY | _____ | _____ | Comments on oral |
| THEATRE | _____ | _____ | spelling: |
| PARTICULAR | _____ | _____ | |
| PHYSICIAN | _____ | _____ | |
| CONSCIENCE | _____ | _____ | |

**Written Spelling Raw Score:** ▢

2. *Written confrontation naming:* Using Cards 2 and 3, have the patient write the names of the following pictured items as they are presented by the examiner.

| | |
|---|---|
| KEY | SEVEN |
| CHAIR | BROWN |
| CIRCLE | RED |
| SQUARE | DRINKING |
| FIFTEEN | SMOKING |

**Raw Score:** ▢

D. *Written Formulation*

1. *Narrative writing:* Present "Cookie Theft" picture (Card 1). "WRITE AS MUCH AS YOU CAN ABOUT WHAT YOU SEE GOING ON IN THIS PICTURE."
Allow patient roughly 2 minutes to write.

Rating (to be circled)

0—No relevant words—Writing is either illegible or paragraphic. There may be some grammatical morphemes, but no recognizable relevant nouns or verbs.

1—Limited number (1 to 4) of relevant words—One or more of the nouns or verbs related to the picture are recognizable (even if misspelled). These may appear as isolated words or embedded in a paragraphic string. There are no legible phrases.

2—One or more phrases—At least one instance of a word combination forming the nucleus of a phrase, e.g., noun plus verb, subject noun plus object noun. There is no sequence of ideas.
OR
Extensive (5 or more) listing of isolated relevant nouns or verbs.

3—Connected ideas—At least two actions or descriptive statements in a connected sequence. No penalty for agrammatism or paraphasic errors.

4—Organized account—Coherent account with only minor paraphasias, grammatical or spelling errors.
OR
Unduly simplified sentences.

5—Normal—Judged normal for patient's premorbid level.

2. *Sentences written to dictation:* Have the patient write these sentences after dictation by the examiner.

A. Score each sentence as follows:
0—Less than 2 words correct
1—At least 2 words correct
2—More than ½ right
3—Correct but laboriously done or paraphrased adequately
4—Normally written

|  | Score |
|---|---|
| a. SHE CAN'T SEE THEM. | ___ |
| b. THE BOY IS STEALING COOKIES. | ___ |
| c. IF HE IS NOT CAREFUL, THE STOOL WILL FALL. | ___ |

Raw Score: ☐

B. Rate paragraphic substitutions
0—conspicuous
1—minor
2—absent

( 26 )

# NOTES

Patient's Name _____ Date of rating _____

Rated by _____

## APHASIA SEVERITY RATING SCALE

0.  No usable speech or auditory comprehension.

1.  All communication is through fragmentary expression; great need for inference, questioning, and guessing by the listener. The range of information that can be exchanged is limited, and the listener carries the burden of communication.

2.  Conversation about familiar subjects is possible with help from the listener. There are frequent failures to convey the idea, but patient shares the burden of communication with the examiner.

3.  The patient can discuss <u>almost all everyday problems</u> with little or no assistance. Reduction of speech and/or comprehension, however, makes conversation about certain material difficult or impossible.

4.  Some obvious loss of fluency in speech or facility of comprehension, without significant limitation on ideas expressed or form of expression.

5.  Minimal discernible speech handicaps; patient may have subjective difficulties that are not apparent to listener.

## RATING SCALE PROFILE OF SPEECH CHARACTERISTICS

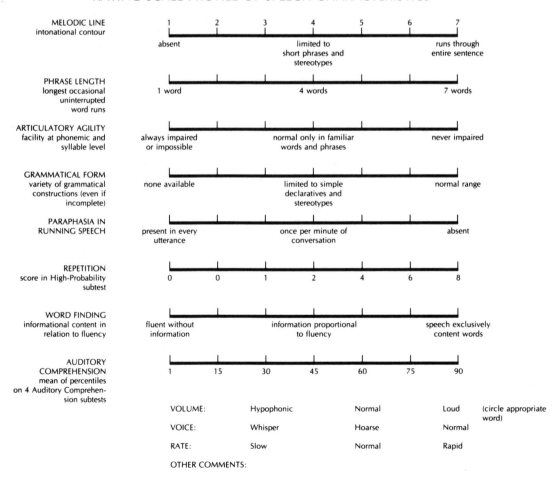

# SUBTEST SUMMARY PROFILE

NAME:                                           DATE OF EXAM:

| | PERCENTILES: | 0 | 10 | 20 | 30 | 40 | 50 | 60 | 70 | 80 | 90 | 100 |
|---|---|---|---|---|---|---|---|---|---|---|---|---|
| SEVERITY RATING | | | 0 | 1 | | | | 2 | | 3 | 4 | 5 |
| FLUENCY | ARTICULATION RATING | | 1 | 2 | 4 | 5 | 6 | | 7 | | | |
| | PHRASE LENGTH | | | 1 | 3 | 4 | 5 | 6 | 7 | | | |
| | MELODIC LINE | | 1 | 2 | 4 | | 6 | 7 | | | | |
| | VERBAL AGILITY | | 0 | 2 | 5 | 6 | 8 | 9 | 11 | 13 | 14 | |
| AUDITORY COMPREHENSION | WORD DISCRIMINATION | 0 | 15 | 25 | 37 | 46 | 53 | 60 | 64 | 67 | 70 | 72 |
| | BODY-PART IDENTIFICATION | 0 | 1 | 5 | 10 | 13 | 15 | 16 | 17 | 18 | | 20 |
| | COMMANDS | 0 | 3 | 4 | 6 | 8 | 10 | 11 | 13 | 14 | 15 | |
| | COMPLEX IDEATIONAL MATERIAL | | 0 | 2 | 3 | 4 | 5 | 6 | 8 | 9 | 11 | 12 |
| NAMING | RESPONSIVE NAMING | | | 0 | 1 | 5 | 10 | 15 | 20 | 24 | 27 | 30 |
| | CONFRONTATION NAMING | | 0 | 9 | 28 | 43 | 60 | 72 | 84 | 94 | 105 | 114 |
| | ANIMAL NAMING | | | 0 | 1 | 2 | 3 | 4 | 6 | | 9 | 23 |
| ORAL READING | WORD READING | | | 0 | 1 | 3 | 7 | 15 | 21 | 26 | 30 | |
| | ORAL SENTENCE READING | | | | | 0 | 1 | 2 | 4 | 7 | 9 | 10 |
| REPETITION | REPETITION OF WORDS | | 0 | 2 | 5 | 7 | 8 | | 9 | | 10 | |
| | HIGH-PROBABILITY | | 0 | 1 | | 2 | 4 | 5 | 7 | 8 | | |
| | LOW-PROBABILITY | | | 0 | 1 | | 2 | 4 | 6 | 8 | | |
| PARAPHASIA | NEOLOGISTIC | 40 | 16 | 9 | 4 | 2 | 1 | | 0 | | | |
| | LITERAL | 47 | 17 | 12 | 9 | 6 | 5 | 3 | 2 | 1 | 0 | |
| | VERBAL | 40 | 23 | 18 | 15 | 12 | 9 | 7 | 4 | 3 | 1 | 0 |
| | OTHER | 75 | 12 | 5 | 3 | 1 | 0 | | | | | |
| AUTOMATIC SPEECH | AUTOMATIZED SEQUENCES | | 0 | 1 | 2 | 3 | 4 | 6 | 7 | | 8 | |
| | RECITING | | | 0 | 1 | | | | | 2 | | |
| READING COMPREHENSION | SYMBOL DISCRIMINATION | 0 | 2 | 5 | 7 | 8 | 9 | | 10 | | | |
| | WORD RECOGNITION | 0 | 1 | 3 | 4 | 5 | 6 | 7 | | 8 | | |
| | COMPREHENSION OF ORAL SPELLING | | | | 0 | 1 | | 3 | 4 | 6 | 7 | 8 |
| | WORD-PICTURE MATCHING | | 0 | 1 | 4 | 6 | 8 | 9 | | 10 | | |
| | READING SENTENCES AND PARAGRAPHS | | 0 | 1 | 2 | 3 | 4 | 5 | 6 | 7 | 8 | 0 |
| WRITING | MECHANICS | 1 | | 2 | | 3 | | 4 | | 5 | | |
| | SERIAL WRITING | | 0 | 7 | 18 | 25 | 30 | 33 | 40 | 43 | 46 | 47 |
| | PRIMER-LEVEL DICTATION | | 0 | 1 | 4 | 6 | 9 | 11 | 13 | 14 | 15 | |
| | SPELLING TO DICTATION | | | | | 0 | 1 | 2 | 3 | 5 | 7 | 10 |
| | WRITTEN CONFRONTATION NAMING | | | | 0 | 1 | 2 | 3 | 6 | 7 | 9 | 10 |
| | SENTENCES TO DICTATION | | | | | | 0 | 1 | 3 | 6 | 8 | 12 |
| | NARRATIVE WRITING | | 0 | 1 | | | 2 | | | 3 | 4 | 5 |
| MUSIC | SINGING | | 0 | 1 | | 2 | | | | | | |
| | RHYTHM | | 0 | 1 | | | | 2 | | | | |
| SPATIAL AND COMPUTATIONAL | DRAWING TO COMMAND | 0 | 6 | 7 | 8 | 9 | 10 | 11 | 12 | | 13 | |
| | STICK MEMORY | 0 | 3 | 4 | 6 | 7 | 8 | 9 | 10 | 11 | 13 | 14 |
| | 3-D BLOCKS | | 0 | 2 | 4 | 5 | 6 | 7 | 8 | 9 | 10 | |
| | TOTAL FINGERS | 0 | 54 | 70 | 81 | 93 | 100 | 108 | 120 | 130 | 141 | 152 |
| | RIGHT-LEFT | 0 | 1 | 3 | 4 | 6 | 8 | 9 | 11 | 14 | 16 | |
| | MAP ORIENTATION | 0 | 2 | 5 | 6 | 9 | 11 | 13 | | 14 | | |
| | ARITHMETIC | | 0 | 2 | 4 | 8 | 11 | 14 | 17 | 21 | 27 | 32 |
| | CLOCK SETTING | 0 | 3 | 4 | 6 | | 8 | 9 | 10 | 12 | | |
| | | 0 | 10 | 20 | 30 | 40 | 50 | 60 | 70 | 80 | 90 | 100 |